Community Mental Health

THERAPY IN PRACTICE SERIES

Edited by Jo Campling

This series of books is aimed at 'therapists' concerned with rehabilitation in a very broad sense. The intended audience particularly includes occupational therapists, physiotherapists and speech therapists, but many titles will also be of interest to nurses, psychologists, medical staff, social workers, teachers or voluntary workers. Some volumes are interdisciplinary, others are aimed at one particular profession. All titles will be comprehensive but concise, and practical but with due reference to relevant theory and evidence. They are not research monographs but focus on professional practice, and will be of value to both students and qualified personnel.

1. Occupational Therapy for Children with Disabilities
   Dorothy E. Penso
2. Living Skills for Mentally Handicapped People
   Christine Peck and Chia Swee Hong
3. Rehabilitation of the Older Patient
   Edited by Amanda J. Squires
4. Physiotherapy and the Elderly Patient
   Paul Wagstaff and Davis Coakley
5. Rehabilitation of the Severely Brain-Injured Adult
   Edited by Ian Fussey and Gordon Muir Giles
6. Communication Problems in Elderly People
   Rosemary Gravell
7. Occupational Therapy Practice in Psychiatry
   Linda Finlay
8. Working with Bilingual Language Disability
   Edited by Deirdre M. Duncan
9. Counselling Skills for Health Professionals
   Philip Burnard
10. Teaching Interpersonal Skills
    A handbook of experiential learning for health professionals
    Philip Burnard
11. Occupational Therapy for Stroke Rehabilitation
    Simon B.N. Thompson and Maryanne Morgan
12. Assessing Physically Disabled People at Home
    Kathy Maczka
13. Acute Head Injury
    Practical management in rehabilitation
    Ruth Garner
14. Practical Physiotherapy with Older People
    Lucinda Smyth et al.
15. Keyboard, Graphic and Handwriting Skills
    Helping people with motor disabilities
    Dorothy E. Penso

16. Community Occupational Therapy with Mentally
    Handicapped Adults
    Debbie Isaac
17. Autism
    Professional perspectives and practice
    Edited by Kathryn Ellis
18. Multiple Sclerosis
    Approaches to management
    Edited by Lorraine De Souza
19. Occupational Therapy in Rheumatology
    An holistic approach
    Lynne Sandles
20. Breakdown of Speech
    Causes and remediation
    Nancy R. Milloy
21. Coping with Stress in the Health Professions
    A practical guide
    Philip Burnard
22. Speech and Communication Problems in Psychiatry
    Rosemary Gravell and Jenny France
23. Limb Amputation
    From aetiology to rehabilitaiton
    Rosalind Ham and Leonard Cotton
24. Management in Occupational Therapy
    Zielfa B. Maslin
25. Rehabilitation in Parkinson's Disease
    Edited by Francis I. Caird
26. Exercise Physiology for Health Professionals
    Stephen R. Bird
27. Therapy for the Burn Patient
    Annette Leveridge
28. Effective Communication Skills for Health Professionals
    Philip Burnard
29. Ageing, Healthy and in Control
    An alternative approach to maintaining the health of older people
    Steve Scrutton
30. The Early Identification of Language Impairment in
    Children
    Edited by James Law
31. An Introduction to Communication Disorders
    Diana Syder
32. Writing for Health Professionals
    A manual for writers
    Philip Burnard
33. Brain Injury Rehabilitation
    A neuro-functional approach
    Jo Clark-Wilson and Gordon Muir Giles
34. Perceptuo-motor Difficulties
    Theory and strategies to help children, adolescents and adults
    Dorothy E. Penso

35. Psychology and Counselling for Health Professionals
    Edited by Rowan Bayne and Paula Nicholson
36. Occupational Therapy for Orthopaedic Conditions
    Dina Penrose
37. Teaching Students in Clinical Settings
    Jackie Stengelhofen
38. Groupwork in Occupational Therapy
    Linda Finlay
39. Elder Abuse
    Concepts, theories and interventions
    Gerald Bennett and Paul Kingston
40. Teamwork in Neurology
    Ruth Nieuwenhuis
41. Eating Disorders
    A guide for professionals
    Simon Thompson
42. Community Mental Health
    Practical approaches to long-term problems
    Steve Morgan

Forthcoming titles

Research Methods for Therapists
Avril Drummond

Stroke: Recovery and Rehabilitation
Polly Laidler

HIV and Aids Care
S. Singh and L. Cusack

Speech and Language Disorders in Children
Dilys A. Treharne

Spinal Cord Rehabilitation
Karen Whalley-Hammell

Community Mental Health

Practical approaches to long-term problems

Steve Morgan

Guy's and Lewisham NHS Trust
Case Management Team
London, UK

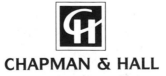

CHAPMAN & HALL

London · Glasgow · New York · Tokyo · Melbourne · Madras

Published by Chapman & Hall, 2–6 Boundary Row, London SE1 8HN

Chapman & Hall, 2–6 Boundary Row, London SE1 8HN, UK

Blackie Academic & Professional, Wester Cleddens Road, Bishopbriggs, Glasgow G64 2NZ, UK

Chapman & Hall Inc., 29 West 35th Street, New York NY10001, USA

Chapman & Hall Japan, Thomson Publishing Japan, Hirakawacho Nemoto Building, 6F, 1–7–11 Hirakawa-cho, Chiyoda-ku, Tokyo 102, Japan

Chapman & Hall Australia, Thomas Nelson Australia, 102 Dodds Street, South Melbourne, Victoria 3205, Australia

Chapman & Hall India, R. Seshadri, 32 Second Main Road, CIT East, Madras 600 035, India

---

Distributed in the USA and Canada by Singular Publishing Group Inc., 4284 41st Street, San Diego, California 92105

First edition 1993

© 1993 Steve Morgan

Typeset in 10/12pt Palatino by Mews Photosetting, Beckenham, Kent
Printed in Great Britain at the University Press, Cambridge

ISBN 0 412 46940 5   1 56593 1386 (USA)

To Mary Vandor
and the memory of John

Contents

Preface   xi
Acknowledgements   xiv

1 Introduction   1

2 Staff structures and support   18

3 Working methods: from theory into practice   46

4 Medical and psychosocial interventions   66

5 Housing   100

6 Finance   123

7 Activities of daily living   141

8 Day care and occupation   159

9 Advocacy and user empowerment   186

10 Conclusions   213

Appendix   218

References   222

Further reading   234

Bibliography   239

Index   245

Preface

The client group referred to as the long-term mentally ill, the persistently severely mentally distressed, the chronically psychotic ill, or people with long-term mental health problems have generally received a poor deal from the traditional psychiatric services. Help has largely rested on custodial and medical treatments. The main focus of rehabilitative approaches has often been dictated by predetermined expectations which are usually set quite low. The assumption is often made that people in this client group are 'treatment resistant' and unlikely to make good use of opportunities to develop personal skills towards restructuring their lives.

Though the emphasis of treatment has often followed medical approaches, and many non-medical people have sought to lay blame on the medical model (as characterized by diagnosis and medical treatments), it would be wrong and greatly over-generalized to follow this line of criticism entirely. In reality, some psychiatrists have been the pioneers and advocates of the diversity of approaches to community support, medical and non-medical. It is they who have often supported the development of other professionals and non-professionals and who often lead the pioneering efforts of research into methods of treatment and support.

Other professionals, including occupational therapists, may learn from the energy and enthusiasm of many psychiatrists, but they also need to be confident in challenging practices that may limit the clients' choice to narrow medical options. We must look to use our own personal skills and professional expertise, with an open mind, towards developing services in the community that are both beneficial and acceptable to the people who receive them, to offer more information and greater opportunities for choice in the way in which they are supported. I propose that this text should be seen as a call for more effective collaboration between professionals in health authorities and local authorities, the voluntary sector, the sources of informal care at home and, above all else, with the clients themselves.

Probably the most radical development in the field of psychiatry, at present, is not the transition from institutional to community care, but the real attempt to address service users' own perceptions of need, encouraging collaboration with the client and the development of the concepts of advocacy and user empowerment. I have specifically included Chapter 9 to address the development of these issues, but I have also attempted to address clients' own perceptions of need as a priority throughout the text. I have also made a number of references to the Personal Strengths Model of Case Management, as developed by Rapp and others at the University of Kansas. My initial introduction to this model of working leads me to believe that it is a most genuine practical effort towards upholding the value of client desires and self-determination as the primary focus of service provision.

As an occupational therapist and a case manager I have experienced a number of different approaches to community support for this client group in a relatively short career. But I advocate the comprehensive case management approach (incorporating the personal strengths model) as a real attempt to focus attention specifically on the needs and wishes of these people.

This approach certainly questions some of the attitudes developed by the traditional stance of established mental health professions, not the least in its promotion of client need above that of profession-based service priorities. But, as an experienced occupational therapist, I can strongly advocate the training and practice of this profession as being directly relevant for this different method of working – particularly the holistic approach, comprehensive assessment, attitude towards engaging with clients, and the focus on personal strengths as well as the strongly developed problem-solving approach.

In proposing a case-management style of response to the provision of mental health services, I am not attempting to draw up a blueprint for changing the fundamental philosophies and roles of the existing professions. What is being proposed is the possibility that a small collective of individuals, from different professional backgrounds but with a common philosophy and interest in the plight of the long-term group, may be organized in a manner that promotes successful service responses. We are particularly concerned here with the needs of clients who are too often termed 'chronic' and 'treatment resistant', people who require services to change their style if they are to be of any relevance.

No one single text, or service approach, will be able to answer all of the questions raised in the work with this client group. Indeed, I am sure many of the questions have not yet been asked! But it is hoped that the text will encourage people to re-examine the professional response towards the needs of the defined client group, to strengthen their views on the meaning of a 'client-centred' approach and possibly help in the development of a healthy and creative attitude towards local community opportunities.

The text is structured to address broad areas of client concern separately – housing, occupation, personal care – but I also aim to address the organizational structure of professional personnel and some of the practical aspects of working methods. It has also been my intention, in most chapters, to follow a particular structure which attempts to separate out the discussion of theoretical issues, practical applications and the case-study materials.

Steve Morgan
Rochester
October 1992

Acknowledgements

I am extremely grateful for the encouragement and advice offered by many people – in particular Alan Beadsmoore, Research Associate with the case management team in North Southwark, for typing the manuscript and regular encouraging discussions; Jean Spencer, the case management teamleader, who reviewed and gave advice on nearly half the text; and each member of the case management team who reviewed individual chapters, namely Cathy Brimelow, Chris May, Noreen Nicholson and Philip Yohuno. Particular thanks are extended to Dr Amanda Poynton, Consultant Psychiatrist, for reviewing sections of the text and for her continued interest and support of the work of the case management team. Peter Ryan at Research and Development for Psychiatry, Martin Kemp of the Lorrimore Centre (voluntary sector day care) and David Shiress and Mark Hopgood (Southwark Housing Resettlement team) have responded with advice in their own areas of expertise.

Special thanks are extended to Charles Rapp and Walter Kisthardt at the University of Kansas for their permission to include the references to the Personal Strengths Model of Case Management and for introducing this model of working in an exciting and enthusiastic manner to British case managers. Special thanks are also extended to Alan Leader and his colleagues at Lambeth Link for reviewing the chapter on advocacy and user empowerment and for their kind permission for the inclusion of their work in the text, helping to illustrate the vital work that is currently undertaken by users and ex-users of mental health services.

Finally, I would like to extend my thanks to Jo Campling, Editor with Chapman & Hall, for valuable comments and guidance through the whole publishing process, thus enabling this text to see the light of day.

1

Introduction

As we approach the twenty-first century I would suggest that the ideas of community care hold the key to providing more responsive mental health services, more suited to the needs and wishes of the individual client. The gradual development and the diversity of initiatives also serves to reflect local circumstances, with an opportunity to engage the collaboration of all relevant people. However, there remains many questions about the economics and the apparent benefits of the shift to community-orientated services (Goodwin, 1989; Warner, 1985).

Community care is not a new idea in the provision of mental health services. As early as 1953 ideas were being expressed about how to make less use of long-term hospital care. There was a growing awareness of the changes affecting people who were spending much of their adult lives in psychiatric institutions – loss of drive, loss of personal identity, loss of dignity as well as a diminishing of ability in daily living skills (Richter, 1984). The emphasis was changing from relying on long-term institutional care towards improving people's rights of self-determination and control over forces affecting them through improved opportunities in the community. Statistically, in the UK, the number of patients occupying mental health hospital beds reached a peak at 143 000 in 1954 (Richter, 1984), falling to 56 200 in 1989 (Ryan, Ford and Clifford, 1991).

The continuing impetus to replace care in large psychiatric hospitals by care through a range of community-based facilities has been maintained through a number of policy initiatives (Ramon, 1988) and different practical innovations. Psychotropic medication, day hospitals, psychiatric units in district general hospitals, community mental health centres and local authority and voluntary sector day centres figure highly in the range of options developed.

However, a major shift in policy will not be met merely by a change of bricks and mortar. Bowden (1991) suggests that 'the move to community care is much more than simply providing the same services to people in a different environment. It is about a change in culture and a fundamental change in the power base of service delivery. It is about negotiating with users and carers what it is that meets their agenda rather than the prescription of service following an assessment.'

Such fundamental changes to the culture and nature of delivering services, particularly for people experiencing long-term severe mental distress, requires a great deal of energy and commitment in a politically motivated and supported atmosphere. The priority of the late 1970s, and through the 1980s, for speeding up the closure of the old mental hospitals, was spurred on by a desire to improve services to the mentally ill. It was also motivated by an attempt to reduce costs. Ryan, Ford and Clifford (1991) produce some bleak figures in reviewing changes between 1978 and 1988, which indicate serious difficulties in transferring financial resources from hospital to community-based services. Expenditure on hospital in-patient services has increased in real terms over this period despite a reduction in numbers of patients, and the percentage expenditure of health and social services on hospital in-patient services has only decreased form 90% to 88% over the same period. In the light of these figures, we need to pay particular attention to the warning of Lavender and Holloway (1988) that 'the will to actually provide community care is fragile, especially when it begins to become clear that the new services are likely to be more expensive, and restrictions on public expenditure become a matter of government strategy'. They go on to suggest that the inevitable financial implications must be challenged by demonstrating the tangible improvements in quality of care for the long-term client.

NOT JUST A QUESTION OF DISCHARGE FROM HOSPITAL

The process of community resettlement was initiated by identifying the less disabled individuals in the long-stay population who may benefit from rehabilitation programmes in the hospital and who may be able to cope with resettlement into a variety of supported accommodation facilities in the community. Indeed, during the 1960s and the 1970s it was felt that the successful rehabilitation of some, and the gradual decline in the number of other long-stay hospital patients through death would naturally lead to less need for such institutions. Other studies (Mann and Cree, 1976) suggested that they were being partially replaced by a new population of people requiring longer term hospital care (new long-stay), some of whom may also be able to benefit from rehabilitation services leading to eventual resettlement back into the community.

However, the experience of long-term severe mental distress, with its accompaniment of multiple needs does not only exist in those who have had long admissions to psychiatric hospitals. A series of studies edited by Wing (1982) into the incidence of long-term mental illness and provision of services in the London Borough of Camberwell suggests that the majority of people experiencing severe difficulties live outside the hospitals, and probably have done so since long before the renewed impetus towards community care. Furthermore, descriptive evidence from McCowan and Wilder (1975) concludes that the main characteristics of institutional living are also much in evidence in the living patterns adopted outside institutions – lack of self confidence, poor self-esteem, lowered motivation, impaired social and personal care skills.

In the USA, Stein and Test (1980) have developed and researched services aimed at maintaining people with long-term persistent mental health problems in the community. Much of this work has formed a basis for the ideas of 'case management' (Ryan, Ford and Clifford, 1991). This involves a case manager having the responsibility for providing an individually tailored package of long-term care in a flexible manner, co-ordinating the input from other services as well as their own clinical interventions. The case manager may also act as an advocate to ensure the clients' real needs are being met, and will be required to monitor the quality of the services being provided. Different models have been developed for the case management functions, which will be discussed more fully in Chapter 2.

The Audit Commission (1986) drew particular attention to the problems of having widely fragmented service provisions for the individual client in the community through many different organizations (health authority, local authority social services and voluntary sector). Subsequent reports (Griffiths, 1988; DoH, 1989, 1991) have attempted to outline methods of addressing the co-ordinated delivery of fragmented services, of which case management has been one potential solution. Whilst this approach has much to offer for severely disadvantaged individuals, there are warning signs that it may be seen as a replacement for the full range of specialist services needed to fulfil many of the complex needs presented (Shepherd, 1990). Clearly, this must be avoided – successful case management relies on adequate provision of a wide range of resources, and an imaginative use of the resources naturally occurring in the community.

Much of the content of this text reflects a 'case management' approach, combining therapeutic practice with the co-ordination of input from a range of service providers. It also provides an opportunity for introducing some of the principle ideas of the personal strengths model of case management (Rapp, 1988). However, it is not intended to extol the virtues of one organizational solution but to look in more detail at the needs of a specific client group and to describe some of the practical options for providing a service to help meet the needs of these individuals.

THEORY INTO PRACTICE

Having identified some of the background to the complex processes underpinning 'community care', I now propose to outline the broad aims of this particular text. A number of writers have already provided us with summaries of the intricate web of policy making in relation to mental health and community care (Ramon, 1988; Ryan, Ford and Clifford, 1991). The subject matter can be approached from a number of perspectives: changing methods of service provision, funding, quality outcome measures, the user perspective, implications for staff training; but whichever theoretical approach is adopted we may still reach the same fundamental conclusion that, in practice, community-based services at least provide a better opportunity to match the real needs of individual consumers more closely. There are widely differing opinions on how this can be achieved, and even doubts cast over the likelihood of its achievement; but the nature of the conflict is now more open and more accessible for debate and negotiation, particularly now that the user movement has a platform to increasingly voice the opinions of the consumers.

A number of recent texts have made serious attempts to bridge the gap from theory to practice in addressing the provision of services for clients experiencing long-term mental health problems in the UK (Lavender and Holloway, 1988; Watts and Bennett, 1991; Pilling, 1991). At a time of ceaseless upheaval in the political context of providing health and social services in Britain, we may be forgiven for being sidetracked into the theoretical frameworks of service provision, to the occasional neglect of detailing what actually happens in the working relationship between client and service provider on a day-to-day basis.

The focus here will be on the practical matters which underlie a 'needs-based, client-centred service for adults experiencing prolonged severe mental distress'. To this end, many of the chapters will follow a specific structure:

- general statements relating to significant issues, including aspects of social policy and reviews of some existing literature;
- detailed personal profiles; and specific case study material to illustrate the chapter content;
- descriptions of practical methods adopted to challenge some of the problems encountered;
- chapter summaries.

It is not intended that the reader should look at this text as a handbook that presents the correct answer to a specific problem. Apart from being extremely presumptuous, such an intention would deny the individuality of the client and the circumstances encountered. Many of the approaches described have met with variable degrees of success or failure (however they may be measured?). What succeeds or fails for one individual may have a completely different outcome for another. The intention is rather one of stimulating creativity when addressing a situation: to encourage a working partnership that is free to attempt different approaches to challenges, that helps a client to use his or her own strengths and creativity, but also allows the professional to explore the scope of his or her own personal and management boundaries when meeting the needs of others. In short, this should be a 'working with' rather than a 'doing for' relationship.

Initially, I wish to address the issue of staffing a community mental health team. If we genuinely wish to achieve a working partnership with the client, we need to look very carefully at the management and working practices of the professional team. Furthermore, the specific client group is often characterized by a difficulty in establishing and maintaining relationships; this, in itself, will influence the working methods of the professionals. In Chapter 2, the emphasis hinges around the value of a close client-worker relationship, to build the confidence necessary to articulate personal needs and begin to work on solutions to the problems identified. The question to be addressed, by professional workers and managers alike, is how to make the best use of staff expertise in meeting the needs of the client group. The answer to this question partly lies in which agenda ultimately takes priority, users' interests or staff efficiency. My own professional background is in occupational therapy and case management, so it is to these that I must turn when examining the debate about staffing issues in multi-disciplinary community teams. The discussion should, however, be equally relevant to other health care professionals.

The systematic processes, based in theory and which usually guide the norms of professional practice, have been well documented. The favoured framework is amply illustrated by the occupational therapy process: assessment, planning, implementation, evaluation (Willson, 1987; Finlay, 1988; Creek, 1990). Chapter three applies the practical bias of this text to the individual components of the framework, illustrating some of the working methods used when attempting to engage, assess, plan and evaluate working with a long-term client group.

The areas of need are highly complex and interrelated for each individual, but for the purposes of clarity they are separated out under different headings. It is this complexity of multiple needs that presents the real challenge to professionals working with the long-term client group, and the personal profiles are presented as a method of recapturing some of that complexity that may be lost to the reader focusing on only one or two chapters in particular.

Medical and psychosocial interventions are discussed in Chapter 4, through a perspective of changed priorities from those prevailing in the institutions. Even a medical model based on the primary functions of diagnosis and prescription of medical treatments has to make some adaptation to survive the transition to a community-orientated service. But this is not an anti-medical model platform. Many of the clients referred to in this text gain a strong sense of security from the relationship with their doctor (GP or psychiatrist) and the prescription of medicine. The case manager will generally spend a significant amount of time facilitating the relationship, monitoring the person's progress and educating clients to increase their own understanding of their mental health and use of medication.

The issue of housing is high on the agenda associated with a move to community care. If we are to successfully run down the large old institutions, we obviously need to provide suitable accommodation for people who suffer from persistent problems. Chapter five examines the question of whether we need to provide highly staffed mini-institutions, or whether we can reasonably start with the premise of providing 'normal' accommodation and assess the variable need for support from this base point. Some form of institutional care is, however, still likely to be necessary for people on restriction orders.

Chapter six examines the political issue of finance. For the individual, the stigma generated by the experience of severe mental distress of a prolonged nature inevitably closes most of the doors that access independent financial means. As a result clients become dependent on budgeting the meagre sums determined by the complex decisions administered through the social security system. For a mental health service the stigma is far less acute, but still evident in a Cinderella relationship alongside the hi-tech medical and surgical demands on the distribution of financial resources.

Chapters 7 and 8 are concerned with personal and day care matters. Western societies place great emphasis on the motivation and ability to address personal appearance,

daily functional requirements and to seek out meaningful productive occupation. Yet this emphasis is often channelled
through criticism rather than the provision of opportunities
to improve standards of achievement, i.e. limited expectations
are often rewarded with limited opportunities.

Finally, Chapter 9 addresses two of the major current issues
in the field of mental health – advocacy and user empowerment. If we genuinely intend to adopt a 'client-centred'
approach, we must take all the opportunities available to
consult and work with the clients of our services. Furthermore, we must work to create opportunities for clients to meet
their own needs. The 'user' movement is here to stay, and
in a practical sense it offers some of the more radically exciting
ideas for service provision. There is a need for all groups
concerned with mental health issues to combine their
knowledge and expertise to address the difficulties faced by
the more disadvantaged clients.

Throughout this text I will be adapting a 'stress-vulnerability'
model to explain the incidence of recurring mental distress. The
basis of this model suggests that distress arises from the interaction of environmental stress factors and biological vulnerability factors with inadequately developed coping mechanisms
for managing the resulting stressful conflict (Onyett, 1992).

LIMITATIONS OF THE TEXT

Many of the issues to be raised could merit an individual
chapter to themselves and each chapter would merit a book
in its own right. Where possible, further references are
suggested to expand the reader's interest. Inevitably, there
must be some significant omissions in the content that follows.
Particular attention is drawn to the expanding minefield of legal
and litigation issues, and to the ever-present need to conduct
research into issues concerned with long-term mental health
problems. The following issues, however, seem to me to
require clearer statements, in the absence of their broader
inclusion in the text.

Physical illness and health promotion

The comparatively inactive lifestyles caused by the limitation dictated by the experiences of severe mental distress, combined with an occasional neglect of personal care and low income to spend on an adequate diet and warmth, indicate that this client group will probably be more susceptible to physical illnesses and disease. Poor housing, heavy smoking and alcohol abuse are strong contributory factors. It is vital that these possibilities should be monitored for fear of misunderstanding the clinical responsibilities – a GP may defer all care to a psychiatrist, but the latter may focus on the clinical speciality to the neglect of physical ailments. Shepherd *et al.* (1981) reported findings of an earlier study of GP practices which suggested that an established group of chronic psychiatric patients was found also to be exhibiting a high incidence of chronic illness. Physical care is, and generally should be, the concern of the GP.

In the case of health promotion, the use of campaigns, advertising and appointments for health checks, e.g. breast screening and cholesterol testing, seem to suggest the need for both awareness of media messages and a motivation to attend for consultations. People suffering from severe mental distress often find difficulty in meeting these particular requirements, which suggests that the people who most need to be targeted are almost always missed by health promotion strategies.

Race and culture

One of the main issues is highlighted by the greater relative proportion of non-white to white people compulsorily detained in government institutions (Willie, Kramer and Brown 1973). One of the main questions is whether the indigenous white population really understand their own use of the terms 'culture' and 'race'. Littlewood and Lipsedge (1989) suggest that 'When looking at another group there is always a tendency to relate psychological difficulties to our own criteria of normality'. The result is often a misinterpretation of the pathological and the cultural.

Fernando (1988) describes how 'in a multi-cultural society where racism is prevalent, cultural issues are not easily differentiated from racial issues'. He concludes that, in Britain, the need to consider the cultural differences in communities is often accepted, but racism is seldom seen as an issue in psychiatric services. It is strongly recommended that we should all seek out some training in order to explore our own mis-understandings before we practise our skills blissfully ignorant of any underlying racist values.

Gender

Only recently have we begun to look beyond the basic statistical differences of gender-related issues and mental health – differences of onset age and prevalence in populations. Bachrach and Nadelson (1988) have helped to highlight many specific needs of women suffering from chronic mental ill-health, including discriminatory practices within and without the mental health services, differing role expectations influencing treatment and outcomes and the very nature of physiological differences requiring specific health care needs, such as regular attention to gynaecological issues.

Carers

'Community Care' is a term adopted relatively recently by professionals to define the changing emphasis of mental health services from an institutional base to a dispersed variety of smaller units of service provision closer to the client's place of residence. For the relatives and friends of people experienc-ing severe mental distress, the notion of community care is one they are all too familiar with, and have been expected to provide, for as long as psychiatric problems have been known. Furthermore, they are also shouldering more of the burden of care with the changes of policy over the last few decades.

The prolonged strain of caring for a severely distressed relative is rarely appreciated by the worker who makes the planned visit with the purpose of assessing the client's situa-tion or providing a specific intervention. It is succinctly encapsulated by a quote from an article in the Observer newspaper : 'It is easy to forget the dimension of time in matters of mental health. A doctor must deal with the patient as he or she is today; health care workers have to sort the crisis of the moment; but a family exhausts itself with fears about the journey of its afflicted member into the dark cave of the future.' (Frankland, 1991.)

Some references are made in the text to support by caring relatives, but it is important to appreciate the roles that they perform and the impact that the suffering of one family member can have on the people close to them (Creer and Wing, 1988; MacCarthy, 1988). Conversely, work has also been carried out to investigate the potential of family dysfunction as a cause of severe distress to one or more family members, particularly around the concept of expressed emotion (Bebbington and Kuipers, 1988). Also some interventions aimed at altering family behaviours in terms of their levels of expressed emotion have shown some positive benefits (Leff and Vaughn, 1985; Falloon *et al.* 1985; Tarrier , 1990).

PROBLEMS WITH DEFINITION

Many attempts have been made to define groups of people who experience severe mental distress, but the complexity of individual difficulties seems to defy the generalizations inherent in definition by a word or short phrase. I would also like to suggest that our need to define the phenomenon we attempt to help causes additional problems of stigma for the client: just as a flight of stairs presents a potential social (as well as physical) disadvantage to the wheelchair user, so the defining of clients in medical terms presents significant social disadvantage through the social stigma and limited expectations that become inherently linked with the words and phrases we have adopted.

Bachrach (1988) suggests that people with long-term mental health problems can be defined in terms of their diagnosis, disability and the duration of their illness. Taken to its extreme, I would suggest this method of categorizing gives rise to statements such as 'long-term chronic schizophrenic' – hardly a good basis from which to build confidence, self-esteem and social networks. Clifford and Craig (1989) propose a further suggestion which follows this system of organization when they suggest that this group includes 'individuals with persistent social and psychological difficulties, as a result of severe psychiatric illness usually of a psychotic nature'. Whilst being more descriptively accurate, this latter statement is still met with disagreement from members of the user movement who claim that terms such as 'persistent', 'psychiatric illness' and 'psychotic' are still loaded against the recipient to create and maintain social stigma.

Medical diagnoses are sometimes abused, resulting in even more denigrating 'slang' to refer to individuals who are already feeling devalued by low self-esteem – 'psycho', 'loony', 'schizo' are but a few of the terms used over many years; 'out to lunch', 'out of your tree', 'the lights are on but nobody is home' are perhaps less brutally stark in their impact but none the less designed to place a devalued status on the individual so described.

Some of the more sympathetic attempts at description have still proved inadequate and raised further objections – 'continuing care' is criticized for ignoring the long periods of time when a person is managing well and not necessarily experiencing the so-called 'symptoms of illness'. For the individual clients discussed in this text 'continuing care' has certain merits; for whatever reasons, some of those individuals apparently do experience symptoms on a persistent basis. Furthermore, the phrase can acknowledge that 'well' (i.e. symptom free) periods are equally significant for developing a working partnership to support the individual in tackling social stigma and personal difficulties that have arisen from dysfunction during periods of illness.

Some members of the user movement prefer to adopt the term 'mental distress'. They acknowledge it too has limitations, but it is strongly preferred to concepts of 'illness' inherent in statements that have grown out of a medical model approach. It is argued that 'illness' and 'care' are terms which explicitly describe a one-way approach of 'doing for', rather than the preferred idea of a partnership 'working with'.

Definition is itself a very limiting concept in that it attempts to encapsulate a very wide-ranging group of individuals, each with specific personal experiences, into one word or a short statement. It is, however, still necessary when we need to focus our attention more specifically on a group of individuals with some collectively shared characteristics. Also, the only true way we can hope to evaluate whether any intervention actually helps is to define the situation first, before we check if it has been resolved in any way.

The group of people I am concerned with in this text are probably already understood by the reader. I will not add to the confusion with my own inadequate attempts to coin the all-encompassing phrase that satisfies all interested parties. Such an exercise would only serve to distract the attention away from the more important function of understanding common characteristics and expressed needs that should more clearly indicate the types of service provision required. Before I outline some of these characteristics, I would like to draw attention to a statement by Pilling (1991) that the 'focus on special needs should not, however, obscure the fact that the basic needs and aspirations of people with long-term illness are no different from those of any other citizen; that is to live with dignity, to have a say in shaping one's own life and to share the experience of life with others'.

GENERAL CHARACTERISTICS OF THE CLIENT GROUP

Their predominant setting is the community, with or without stable accommodation. They include some people who have previously spent long periods of time in hospital; others have had regular contact with formal psychiatric services over long periods of time, including many short hospital admissions; and in a few cases distress has been experienced over a long time but there may have been little or no previous contact with formal services.

In psychiatric terms, the majority of the clients have been described as suffering a psychotic illness – usually schizophrenia. They are often also characterized by a long history with multiple diagnoses, reflecting both the complexities of the clinical picture and the difficulties in achieving a consensus of opinion in an imprecise speciality.

Individuals have experienced difficulty in establishing and maintaining personal relationships, often resulting in poor networks of support and social isolation. Family relationships can vary from offering the very highest quality support to being highly critical, rejecting and intensifying the wider felt social stigma associated with society's views of severe mental disturbance.

They have complex multiple needs, including a high incidence of physical ill health resulting from serious social and economic disadvantages in addition to the personal disadvantages implicit in the experience of severe distress.

As will be apparent to the reader from the discussion above, there is no 'typical' individual who reflects all of the complex characteristics of a defined client group. In this text, case material will be presented in two distinguishable forms:

1. Personal profiles – designed to emphasize the complex multiple difficulties faced by an individual in this client group (not just problems associated with the specific chapter content).
2. Case studies – designed to focus on the issues related to the content of the particular chapter rather than the individual person.

The following personal profile is included at this point to give a practical example of the multiple needs expressed by individuals in this client group.

PERSONAL PROFILE

Mary is a 56-year-old widow living alone in a one-bedroom housing association flat on the first floor of a terraced house. Her first admission to a psychiatric hospital lasted for 20 years from 1955, when she was only 20 years of age. Diagnosed as suffering chronic schizophrenia, Mary became institutionalized at a time when the hospital population was declining rapidly, soon after the discovery and use of psychotropic medication. She generally acknowledges some value from oral and intramuscular medication, despite the functionally inhibiting effects of a permanent extra-pyramidal tremor and stereotyped limb movements (tardive dyskinesia) and the continuous experience of auditory hallucinations.

In 1975 Mary was able to benefit from the progressive policy of closing the long-stay psychiatric institutions. She and her husband were discharged shortly after their marriage to set up home in the flat she still occupies (though this may have been more to do with expectations of the marriage than hospital closure policy). They were able to share the flat until his death in 1990. Mary describes how they were able to support each other during their 15 years together by assuming traditional roles – she took responsibility for shopping and cooking while her husband managed their welfare benefits and bills. Services support was offered to them by way of community psychiatric nurse and district nurse visits to administer depot injections and her husband's insulin injections. However, during much of their time together the furnishing and décor of the flat became progressively neglected.

Mary also neglected her own appearance and personal hygiene at this time, wearing soiled and grubby clothing, neglecting to heat the flat during the winter period and failing to wash, resulting in the appearance of ingrained dirt in her skin.

Mary experiences a wide range of physical complaints. Weight loss is quite marked through poor attention to diet since her husband's death. Thyrotoxicosis has resulted from an overactive thyroid gland with accompanying speeding up of her metabolism; abnormal protrusion of the eyes (exophthalmos), excessive growth of facial hair and a possible contribution to the extrapyramidal tremor may be the result. The thyrotoxicosis may also contribute towards the aforementioned weight loss. The exophthalmos has also played a part in the development of a progressive infection and ulceration of her eyes, which becomes further aggravated by occasional periods of heavy smoking. Despite these complex physical complaints, Mary experiences difficulty in using appointments with primary or hospital care services to monitor the situation.

The neglect of personal care and the condition of the flat became a marked feature over the 10 months following the death of her husband, The décor took on a mixed hue of yellows and browns, with widespread fungal growth from the damp. The flat became cluttered with decaying food, furniture and clothing, and the ash and cigarette ends progressively over-filled the ash trays and other neglected items of crockery. To compound the decaying state of the flat, a flood from the flat above resulted in a widespread peeling of ceiling and wallpaper and a more serious collapse of the kitchen ceiling.

Social isolation is a persistent feature since the death of her husband. Though a sister-in-law visits occasionally,

Mary tends to shun any consideration of social contact. She continues to express the wish that her husband should return, occasionally acknowledging his death but frequently experiencing his presence through her hallucinatory experiences. Her response to other people can vary from verbal hostility to periodic short engagements in conversation of a repetitive nature – only apparently receptive to a small number of topics at any one time before needing to suddenly terminate contact.

Positive characteristics

Mary is relatively financially secure and generally manages to follow advice on financial matters. She receives a widow's pension on a weekly basis and would be entitled to further welfare benefits. She also has sufficient savings from her own and her husband's accounts. Mary usually manages to cash her benefits order book and pays bills that arrive through the post. She has difficulty in understanding the reasoning of some financial circumstances but follows advice and help for paying or applying for rebates.

Mary is consistent in her expressed desire to continue living in her current flat. She requests support to help her stay at home rather than move to more supported accommodation but tends to be inconsistent in allowing access to the flat to meet her requests for help – she generally allows access to help with her physical health needs but resists access to help with personal and domestic care, despite previously acknowledging a need for such help.

She uses the local shopping street and market for some of her needs and for cashing her order book at the post office.

Mary's statements of need are:

- redecoration and refurbishment of her flat to make it habitable;
- deceased husband should return to the flat to help her cope at home;
- regular medication to help her stay out of hospital;
- help to wash dishes and clean the flat;

- help to administer eye drops to control the eye infections;
- help to control the rapid growth of facial hair.

Some of Mary's specific needs will be addressed through case study material in the relevant chapters of this text.

2

Staff structures and support

Any discussion of the staffing of a community mental health service must begin with the basic premise that it will be constituted from a disparate range of people and agencies, professional and non-professional, geographically separated, performing structured and unstructured tasks. The quality of communication between the constituent parts may also be variable, they may well operate from a basis of very different motivations and lay claim to their different rights for recognition through statements of philosophy and operational policy.

Somewhere in the middle of this divergent group of people will be an individual client, identified as the person who has been suffering from the experiences of long-term mental distress and for whom each of the caring members of the 'community' will be staking a claim to know what they need in the form of 'help'.

In reality, the people who most clearly know what they 'want' are the individual clients themselves. This will also include a knowledge of what they 'need'. In view of the frequent difficulties associated with developing and maintaining relationships, it is likely that they will prefer an adequate level of communication and teamwork to be performed by those claiming to be offering help.

Most of the health care professions will make their own claims to offer a service to this specific client group, stating the significant value of their core skills, whether offered from a uni- or multi-professional standpoint. However, if we consider a defined client group to have specific needs, the multi-disciplinary team is generally viewed as the cornerstone of specialist service provision (Øvretveit, 1989). Within this chapter I propose to evaluate the different options for organizing the staffing of services intended to meet the needs of a long-term client group.

The development of the multi-disciplinary team has recently been accompanied by the phrase 'skills mix'. In its pure form, this would refer to the balance of different professions within a team, each offering their distinctive core skills and sharing some of the common administrative tasks. Some writers have suggested we need to look further, to shared skills, to personal skills and to the benefits accrued from specialist postgraduate training opportunities. Meteyard (1990) indicates that team-work can accomplish more than the sum of its individual parts, with organizations often failing to capitalize on the full potential of their individual workers.

However we may view the concept of teamwork in multi-disciplinary teams, there is still the inherent danger of building the notion of a service in a vacuum, with the individual client slotted into the established pattern as an afterthought. Most services would claim to be needs-based and client-centred, but very few traditional mental health services would be able to make a claim to meet the complex multiple needs presented by this specific client group. Miller (1988) also discusses a range of criticisms made against the formal services by the army of informal carers who provide the backbone of support to suffering relatives and friends.

How the skills of support are delivered to those in need, and the question of 'Who does what best for whom?' are the subjects of intense ongoing debate.

In the professional context, the value of specific training and the core skills of each profession must be recognized and remain vitally important. But in a client-centred context they must be seen in a realistic light – the person with a long history of severe mental distress and fragmented relationships will find great difficulty separating out his or her own needs on professionally defined lines and establishing a close working relationship with each individual professional who deals with special areas of need. In this case, it is more likely that the person will respond to one professional as a focal point for discussing wants, needs and the wider range of services that may be available.

The style of working is more often referred to as *keyworking* but can itself, take on many guises and titles. What will be discussed subsequently are the different methods of performing such a role. It may require special postgraduate training or it could evolve into a new profession, but it is not meant to be presented as a blueprint for altering or subsuming the training and experience of the wide range of existing workers. Contrary to the fears of existing professionals that their professional identity and role is about to be taken over, this is a specialist area of practice that may appeal to individual workers from a wide variety of backgrounds and experience. Furthermore, a particular concept of case management will be evaluated as a more specialist form of keyworking, which emphasizes a need for smaller case-loads in order to undertake a more intensive and comprehensive range of functions with each individual.

Much of the debate, in the professions, about styles of delivering individual community support has tended to focus on the potential loss of role and identity for the support workers, or it has focused rather specifically on the semantics around new job titles, with little consideration for the substance of the service to be offered. It is my contention that most of the issues raised by the objections could be managed through the setting up of adequate, if not elaborate, systems of staff support and supervision. Such systems may even justify the more contentious issue of using the considerable resource of experienced, though unqualified, support staff, many of whom are highly regarded by individuals in the client group and viewed with less suspicion about their motives and loyalties.

PROVIDERS OF SUPPORT

The potential sources of help and support in the community are many and varied (see Figure 2.1). They may be seen as forming a multicoloured patchwork. Unlike the traditional large mental hospital where the range of services could be co-ordinated under a single organizational structure, the nature of community services is that of sporadic growth in differently organized, coexisting structures. Inevitably this leads to problems of communication and co-ordination on a far greater scale than previously experienced in the institutions. This chapter will mainly be concerned with only a part of Figure 2.1, specifically within the health authority sector, but wider

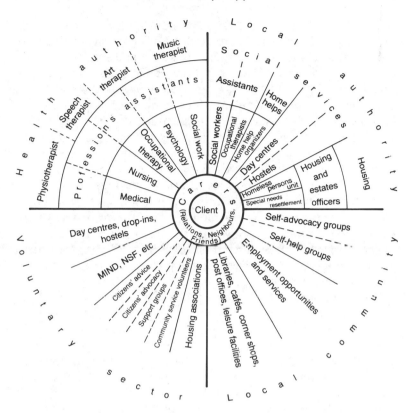

Figure 2.1 Providers of support.

problems of communication will be magnified when we consider the whole picture.

The models for developing the professional multi-disciplinary practice in the community grew largely out of the co-operation of the different professions working together within the hospital settings, but it has been extended in the community to implement more innovative practice through sharing tasks and skills across professional boundaries. This latter move has met with some criticism and resulted in the professions looking more introspectively at their own skills base. Such a move also has an element of inevitability, both from the perspective of individual professionals wishing to extend the boundaries of their own skills and from the greater organizational demands imposed by the community setting as opposed to the more insular hospital setting.

One exception to the rule has been the role of the psychiatrist. Patmore and Weaver (1991) highlight some of the dilemmas perceived around the position of a psychiatrist *vis-à-vis* a multi-disciplinary community support team, particularly with regard to the historical position of influence and authority occupied by consultant psychiatrists. Whether having a direct or indirect working relationship with a team, the consultant is often perceived as the manager or director of the team. The greater statutory responsibilities afforded to the position make it impossible for a consultant to engage in any degree of role blurring within the team, though there may be scope for more flexibility in short-term contracts for junior doctors (depending on their specific training needs and the frequent demands placed on them to cover other clinics).

From the perspective of the other health care professions, there is also an amount of scepticism expressed regarding the forging of close links with a consultant psychiatrist. They are often seen as carrying valuable 'political clout', but concerns are still expressed that this will be accompanied by a domination of the team's practice, with the possibility of undermining innovative methods of working – particularly any attempt to move away from conventional professional roles. After all, chronic mental illness can still be seen to occupy a central role for justifying the medical model of clinical practice through the core functions of diagnosis, based on the signs and symptoms of illness and medical treatments. But this view of the consultant psychiatrist as restricting innovation also needs to be balanced by an acknowledgement that some psychiatrists have been the instigators of radical change and are at the forefront of researching new developments well beyond the limited scope attributed to a medical model such as the one mentioned above.

The position accredited to unqualified staff as a part of the professional agency provision of support is only recently becoming recognized in the UK. We need to look to the experience of the US case management projects, and again we find differing opinions in the validity of their roles. Rapp and Wintersteen (1989) have concluded, from a study of twelve projects, that much of the support required by people suffering from long-term mental health problems can be undertaken by 'para-professionals' and 'batchelor-level professionals', under the close supervision of fully qualified staff. Bachrach (1989) presents evidence from different projects to show how, in some cases, the philosophy of Rapp and Winterseen is being practised, but other projects emphasize the nature of the work as a clinical entity requiring the tasks to be performed by fully qualified health professionals.

The debate continues, but it would appear that unqualified staff with good experience and support can perform the type of support requested by clients, often from a position less cluttered by the baggage of training, role conformity and inter-personal rivalries. However, with the unqualified role goes lower status and lower pay. This should not be seen primarily as the cheap option for providing an expensive service or, once again, service needs would be placed before client needs, possibly only justified by a short-term economic policy.

Informal care, whether through immediate carers, the voluntary sector or local community resources, is the major source of support for many people experiencing persistent severe distress. However, it is often felt to be undervalued by the formal services and generally continues to be left unsupervised (as seen by the formal services meaning of 'support and supervision'). Sometimes the existence of informal care is used negatively by the formal services as a way of eliminating or reducing the option of support within priorities set by the finite level of resources available. So the person living alone may well be seen as a higher priority than those living with family or friends, even before the circumstances of need and potential domestic conflict and stress are considered.

Clearly, the potential for support in the community is vast, but the immense need for good communication and networking must be addressed to make full use of what is available. The need for good quality support and supervision also extends way beyond the boundaries of individual professional line management. The government White Paper 'Caring for People' (1989) specifically emphasizes the need for developing networks of informal care with a flexible approach, enabling services to work alongside, and support, the relatives and carers often at the front line of care.

SHOULD THE EMPHASIS REMAIN ON 'CORE' SKILLS?

One of the mainstays of the concept of 'professionalism' is the ability to uphold the identity of each profession through a claim to unique skills requiring unique training. Such as identity is defined by its core skills (Onyett, 1992) and defended by the exclusion zone of its language (jargon). The changing management styles of the late 1980s and the early 1990s require each profession to be more clear in the definition of its unique skills and expertise in order to promote more efficient use of resources. Indeed, Brown (1991) goes as far as to suggest the 'survival' of a profession depends on its competitive edge. The occupational therapy profession must either clearly identify those functions which only it can perform or it must provide a cheaper operational generic service than other professions. Failure to achieve either of these requirements may ultimately result in the merging of occupational therapy into a larger profession, resulting in an almost complete loss of identity.

Not to raise the anxiety of occupational therapists too high, the above view can be judged against the report of the Audit Commission (1986) which suggests that the OTs are in many ways central to the implementation of community care, that these skills are too important to be in only limited supply and that all OTs should be encouraged to provide the specialist skills which only they can perform, namely functional assessment, selection of aids and design of adaptations.

Whilst the Audit Commission statement indicates a broad range of skills, occupational therapy, as a profession, has long experienced an internal struggle to define itself adequately. Like the other professions, it has required its practitioners to contribute to the ongoing debate of defining skills. Joice and Coia (1989) have used a previously established framework of four classes of skills common to each discipline in a multi-disciplinary team: required and restricted practices related to qualifications, core skills, basic common skills and special interest skills acquired through further education.

In the cases of occupational therapy, Joice and Coia (1989) suggest that the formal assessment of functional capabilities in the area of activities of daily living should become a restricted practice (though it is not defined as such yet). The core skills are defined as the use of selected activity as a treatment medium, activity analysis and the assessment and treatment of functional capabilities. The basic common skills, shared by all professions, are seen as the knowledge of psychopathology and models of psychiatry, observation, interviewing, counselling, education, group therapy and communication and management skills. Special interests are identified by the examples of psychodrama, psychoanalytic therapy, analytic art and transactional analysis. (For further discussions of the specific skills of occupational therapists see Brown, 1991; Thorner, 1991.)

One of the problems of debating the skills specific to a single profession is that you may gain a degree of consensus within a profession but multi-professional discussions rarely, if ever, reach any clear conclusions. With the exception of a few statutory requirements, such as prescribing and administering medications or sectioning under the mental health legislation, there will always be a degree of argument about who is capable of performing which skills (Onyett, 1992). However, Joice and Coia (1989) do suggest that if practices could be restricted by profession there may be a greater quality of care offered to patients through specialist professionals. Professional responsibilities may become clearer with more clearly delineated areas of clinical practice, and there may be a reduction in role insecurity and role envy between professions. Loss of role and identity appear to be frequent arguments against any suggestion of sharing or blurring roles in multi-disciplinary teams.

Where does this leave the individual client experiencing long-term mental health problems after the professions have clarified their professional roles among themselves? I would suggest that this still leaves them confused and distanced from the whole range of services they may require to meet their complex multiple needs. They are still likely to be left in need of an advocate with knowledge of the system and its access points.

The uni-professional team, practising its restricted skills and basic common skills, tends to perform a specialist function, but to a generic client group. Just as the hospital-based psychiatric occupational therapy department will offer a specialist service to patients with chronic and acute conditions across a wide range, so, too, will a community psychiatric occupational therapy service. The corollary to this may also be equally valid, that the specialist client group with a wide range of needs must require a more generically operating worker to establish a relationship, help to assess strengths and weaknesses and support access to the workers performing the core skills.

The purists among the different professions still advocate a multi-disiplinary team made up of representatives of each profession and practising their own professional skills for each client referred to the service. This system is likely to promote the clarity of each profession but may continue to deny the personal qualities and experience that each individual may bring to a team. We still need to overcome our fears, the perceived threat in the notion that 'the team is greater than the sum of its parts'.

Craik (1991) examines recent concerns expressed within the profession about occupational therapists leaving to become general managers and care managers. It is viewed by some as a loss of numbers and talent for such a small profession. But she argues that this need not be seen as a loss: 'Rather, it allows an opportunity for the profession to mature and grow in its ability to affect decision-making.' The scope of the profession can be extended by meeting the new challenges facing health and social services organizations. OTs can help to create policy and be proactive in decision-making.

Craik suggests that introspection and self-criticism have served to strengthen the foundations of the occupational therapy profession but should not extend to stifling opportunities to broaden the horizons of individual OTs or the profession as a whole. Murdoch (1988) also advocates the positive aspects of extending personal skills across professional boundaries to a level that suits the worker, the client, the employer and the available resources. This is seen as a practical way of extending the opportunities available to the individual client.

THE KEYWORKER IN MULTI-DISCIPLINARY TEAMS

I have already suggested that this method of teamwork grew out of the experience of co-operation perceived between professionals in institutional settings; but, from the discussion outlined by Øvretveit (1989), it is possible to list tangible reasons for organizing staff into multi-professional teams:

- to ensure that clients receive a service which is better than the one which they would receive if each profession and agency were helping them independently;
- to promote a better understanding of the special skills of each profession and of the resources available, through working more closely with other professions in the team;
- to achieve better planning proposals from teams and improve their ability to identify gaps in services;
- to ensure easier workload management and to establish common priorities across professions;
- to offer specialist support from different professions with common interests.

The implication is that a multi-disciplinary team will include representatives of each profession, capable of performing core skills and sharing the basic common skills in order to achieve the tasks set out for the team. But to meet the requirements of the specific client group and for the functions of the team to focus through one individual, we have the organizational arrangement known as the **keyworker**.

Meteyard (1990) defines the keyworker simply as 'an identified person who is charged with a defined responsibility towards a specific service user'. The range of activities that a keyworker may perform on behalf of an individual client may be many and varied:

- providing access to the services of other team members;
- problem-solving;
- explaining clients' needs and advocating for them;
- explaining the intricacies of the system to the client;
- preparing necessary referral arrangements;
- supporting service users through specialist core skills;
- advocating for new services.

Essentially, the individual worker will hold clinical and managerial responsibilities for the people to whom they are designated as keyworker as well as providing core skills to the users of the service when another team member (keyworker) requests the input. The finer details of the role would be determined by the operational policies agreed for the particular service.

Ultimate responsibility for decision-making regarding the service that can be offered to an individual client should remain a team function. The decisions should be made through its clinical and policy-making forums, leaving the individual keyworker to perform the co-ordination and monitoring of the collective work of the team. Such co-ordinating and monitoring functions should be seen as basic common skills and can thus be undertaken by members of any profession (Watts and Bennett, 1991).

The concept of the keyworker in a multi-disciplinary team contrasts sharply with the same title used in the uni-profession team. For example, the occupational therapist in the former acts on behalf of the whole team, where each of the profession's representatives share a defined interest in the client. The occupational therapist in a community occupational therapy team will disuss a client in team meetings but is more likely to be the 'sole worker' from that team directly involved with the client, while other team members, with their own client caseload, take responsibility for the direct work.

A significant difficulty in performing such a range of functions in a multi-disciplinary team can arise if the initial organization and management of the team is not clearly thought out: different members of a team may be distinguished by different training, different professional and line management loyalties, different ethical principles and different lines of accountability; they may work in one or several teams, work full-time or part-time in the team, have different degrees of autonomy, operate under different referral procedures, have different procedures for sharing information with service users and work on different rates of pay (Meteyard, 1990). To provide an efficiently co-ordinated service to a client can become a very difficult task if the background of professional differences outlined above has not been addressed through service implementation and team-building processes.

Reid (1988) suggests that multi-disciplinary work has its value for promoting co-operation and communication between professions; but she highlights the predominance of teams being set up in either health authority or social services department organizations with little cross-fertilization. Consequently, a keyworker in a particular team has relatively good access to health workers or social care workers, but not both. Whilst occupational therapy is frequently heralded as one of the few professions with personnel in both structures, the continued call for more communication between OT colleagues seems to fall short of meeting the multiple needs of the specific client group with experiences of persistent severe mental distress. In these particular cases, the keyworker role may also be hampered by the compromise necessary to offer a co-ordinating function to some and core skills function to many others.

It is with these limitations in mind, and as a response to the complex multiple needs of this particular client group, that the concept of the 'case manager' has developed.

THE CASE MANAGER IN MULTI-DISCIPLINARY TEAMS

The first few words must take the form of a cautionary note, as this is an area that could potentially become depleted by arguments over semantics which would bypass the more important content of what these roles have to offer the person suffering from long-term mental health problems. Many argue against the title 'case manager' on the grounds that the person receiving a service objects to being referred to as a 'case' whose life is 'managed' by others. In my own experience, no client has yet made such objections, even if I bring the subject up for discussion openly; one client did, however, reverse the terminology by referring to me as the 'case' who came to visit him.

I sympathize strongly with the statements about the inadequacy of the title, but it is now becoming more confused within a plethora of titles, including care management and the care programme, emanating from government policy statements. Table 2.1 outlines the basis of the different

Table 2.1 Terminology

Functions	Case management	Care Management	Care programme
Defining the client	'Where individual needs are complex or significant levels of resources are involved.' Multiple need clients who: (i) may have behavioural difficulties (ii) do not easily engage with services (iii) might otherwise remain in hospital.	Interface between primary and secondary care. Clients in need of care who have previously been hospitalised but who are not receiving a care programme.	'For people with a mental illness including dementia referred to specialist psychiatrist services '(HC(90)23). Priority group likely to be those acute or long-stay clients for whom better co-ordination of existing services is likely to provide adequate community support.
Assessment	Comprehensive, in-depth assessment of individual needs for health and social care	Broad overview in order to establish eligibility for services and to clarify priorities for package of care. May refer for specialist assessment in priority areas.	? Broad overview in order to establish eligibility for services and to clarify priorities for package of care.

Developing the care plan	Overall responsibility of case manager in co-operation with local services, user and carer.	Overall responsibility of care manager in co-operation with keyworker.	Overall responsibility of consultant psychiatrist in co-operation with hospital care team and social services.
Package of care	Negotiated by case manager in co-operation with local services, user and carer. Case manager provides ongoing co-ordination.	Commissioned by care manager on basis of overall assessment plus additional specialist assessment where appropriate. Keyworker may have ongoing co-ordination role.	Negotiated by hospital care team prior to discharge, in co-operation with local services. keyworker may have ongoing co-ordination role.
Provision of direct service	Depending on availability of local services, may well include significant amount of direct case management work with client.	No input by care manager. Direct care provided by specified services included in package of care, plus keyworker where appropriate.	Provided by services included in agreed package of care. May include direct input from keyworker.
Monitoring and review	Stays with case manager.	Could stay with care manager or transfer to keyworker.	Could stay with consultant psychiatrist or transfer to keyworker.

(Source: Ryan, Ford and Clifford (1991) *Case Management and Community Care*, p. 34. Published with kind permission.)

terminology currently being used. In brief, we may refer to a simplified outline of the functions as follows:

- Keyworker: the identified individual from a team (uni- or multi-disciplinary) who will provide the focal point for service provision from that team and link with other potential service providers for the individual (Meteyard, 1990).
- Case Manager: a similarly identified role to the keyworker, with a more comprehensively addressed degree of responsibility for assessment, potential direct service provisions and co-ordination of other service providers across the full range of individual client needs and strengths (Ryan, Ford and Clifford, 1991; Onyett, 1992).
- Care Manager: has an identified duty to make a broad overview assessment of the community needs of an individual client, calling for specialist assessments in priority areas, develop the package of care and commission specific services, which may or may not involve direct service provision. Review may remain with the care manager or be shared with others, such as case managers or keyworkers (Ryan, Ford and Clifford, 1991; Allen, 1990).
- Care Programme: a process established for psychiatric patients in hospital to ensure discharge to adequately assessed and developed care. It requires close co-operation of health care and social care providers in hospital and in the community. Responsibility for developing the plan lies with the consultant psychiatrist, but subsequent monitoring may remain here or transfer to others, perhaps case managers or keyworkers (Ryan, Ford and Clifford, 1991; Onyett, 1992).

At this point we need to look at the practical implications of the concept of care management perhaps that can enhance the access to services for people suffering from persistent distress. I have suggested above that even the keyworker principle in multi-disciplinary teams presents limitations for people with more severe multiple difficulties, since it is likely that case-load size, time and multiple demands on the keyworker's job may limit the intensity of the work and attention to detail that may be required by people in this client group. For this reason, case management has been developed according to a number of different models, predominately to consider how to shape a service to meet individual requirements and take responsibility for ensuring the clients receive the services they want and need.

The brokerage model is an administrative response (Bachrach, 1989) with a philosophy similar to that of key-working, stressing the need for the co-ordination of service elements to assist people in gaining access to the resources they need. This particular model of case management limits the numbers of functions performed and enables larger case-load sizes. It appears to be a popular model for the wholesale restructuring of existing services particularly favoured by local authority social services departments at present.

The 'strengths' and 'clinical' models of case management are interactional responses, stressing the central importance of the client–care manager relationship and the subsequent need for small case-loads to enable intensive work to be invested in the relationship (Rapp and Wintersteen, 1989; Kanter, 1989).

The six principles of the strengths model of case management (Rapp, 1988; Rapp and Kisthardt, 1991) are as follows.

1. The focus of the helping process is upon the clients' strengths, interests, abilities, competencies and not upon their deficits, weaknesses or problems.
2. All clients have the capacity to learn, grow and change.
3. The client is viewed as the director of the case management helping process.
4. The client–case manager relationship becomes a primary and essential partnership.
5. The case management helping process takes on an outreach perspective, occurring more in the community than at the office base of a mental health resource.
6. The entire community is viewed as an oasis of potential resources for clients rather than as an obstacle. Naturally occurring resources are considered as a possibility before institutionalized or segregated mental health services.

The desired consequences of these principles are that:

- a strengths perspective should promote a strongly individualized view of the client and his/her specific circumstances;
- a strengths perspective should facilitate the growth of partnerships rather than adversaries;

- a strengths perspective should foster user empowerment.
- a strengths perspective should seek to blend and unify the goals of the client, the service provider and the local community.

The close relationship between client and case manager is described as the element which provides the buffer of support during anxious times: it helps to prevent or reduce the intensity of symptoms and it supports the client's confidence to challenge the difficulties they experience (Rapp, 1988). Kanter (1988) suggests that this type of relationship manifests all of the dynamics encountered in psychotherapy but without the constraints of the parameters which bind the formal psychotherapy relationship. He suggests a number of characteristics of the relationship which can transcend the differences of ideology, professional discipline and the setting for the work:

- clients experience significant impairments in managing the activities of daily living and social relationships;
- case managers act as intermediaries between the client and the environment;
- case managers act as 'travelling companions, easing the loneliness of the client's journey';
- case managers respond to client needs in a variety of settings;
- necessary, normal and constructive forms of client dependency are managed;
- the majority of interventions have a public dimension, requiring the case manager to surrender the privacy of the work base or office.

The emphasis on relationship factors closely matches the underlying philosophy of the occupational therapy profession (and probably each of the other health care professions). Lloyd and Maas (1991) discuss the key element of the relationship between the occupational therapist and the client, suggesting that the outcome of interventions depends on pulling together the separate components of client, therapist, therapeutic relationship, the activity and the context. Brown (1991) also emphasizes the importance of the relationship factors when discussing the distinctive aspects of the occupational therapy profession. He notes that in contrast to some of the other professions, occupational therapy carries no statutory powers. He concludes that this position requires the occupational therapist to invest more effort in the relationship to make the service more attractive by fitting interventions to needs and by promoting greater empowerment to clients of the service.

The functions of a case management approach are widely discussed in the literature (Ryan, Ford and Clifford, 1991; Kanter, 1989; Bachrach, 1989; Witheridge, 1989). Kanter suggests that 'moving beyond a limited view of the case manager as a systems coordinator, service broker, or supportive companion, . . . [they] are concerned with all aspects of their patients' physical and social environments, including housing, psychiatric treatment, health care, entitlements, transportation, families, and social networks'. Witheridge, however, preferring to use the term 'assertive community treatment worker', suggests that it is very difficult to draw up a specific job description because the functions vary from client to client and from day to day. The constant in the equation would be the defined client group, but the roles performed may include any or all of the following:

- identifying members of the target population;
- engaging new participants;
- conducting assessments;
- planning interventions;
- assuming ultimate responsibility for developing individualized packages of care;
- assertive outreach mode of working;
- providing *in vivo* assistance and training;
- arranging psychiatric and other medical services;
- providing inter-agency resource brokering and advocacy;
- developing community resources;
- facilitating readmissions to hospital, if necessary;
- working in partnership with families and other carers.

It is widely accepted that the case manager would take on a wider range of functions with the individual client and carry more responsibility for assuring the wide range of needs are met, carefully monitored and reviewed than would the key-worker. In contrast to the brokerage model, case managers acting through the personal strengths or clinical models will find themselves actively involved in a range of clinical functions. As a result of the width and intensity of the role, many writers stress the need for case-load sizes to be kept relatively low – Harris and Bergman (1988) note that service planners require 1–20 to 1–40, but the reality from studies suggests 1–12 to 1–15 because case managers frequently find themselves filling the gaps in treatment services by providing needed clinical services themselves.

These models are also characterized by a mode of working referred to as 'assertive outreach', a term which can be the subject of conflicting interpretations. In some cases it is given a negative connotation, the criticism being one of infringing on personal liberty by constantly chasing a client who has no desire to engage in any services. It is easy to see how such a negative viewpoint has materialized, because the clients primarily targeted for case management are often described as 'treatment resistant' or 'persistently avoiding or dropping out of services'. In practice, it has generally been found that few people look to resist a service that is packaged and presented to genuinely offer what they might want. They do, however, resist services that their own experience tells them do not suit their wants and needs.

If we distinguish the negative approach as being 'aggressive outreach', the more positive meaning of 'assertive outreach' stresses the value of meeting the client at preferred venues – at home, at work, at a café, in the park. This highlights the public dimension of the relationship suggested above by Kanter which will be discussed more fully in the section on 'Engagement' in Chapter 3.

The emphasis of the work, for the individual case manager, tends to be on the basic common skills described earlier in the chapter, but with an acknowledgement that the person brings to the team identified core skills and personal commitment beyond the normal scope of a single profession. It is possible for the individual to extend expertise beyond professional training, through further training, experience and adequate support and supervision. It is possible to continue acknowledging one's own core skills and to have those respected within a team, without having to be limited in scope to performing these skills, to ensure that clients have access to good quality services.

No one single profession can lay a claim to monopolize the skills of case management because individuals from each of the professions can bring a mix of philosophies, training and personal experience to enrich a team set up for the purpose of supporting an identified client group in the community. Only by sharing all these ingredients can the team achieve the position of being greater than the sum of its parts.

Community psychiatric nurses and social workers occasionally lay claim to be already doing the work or express fears that a new team would endanger their posts. In reality this is far from the case as the existing professions tend to work with generic case-loads. Certainly, no single profession could lay claim to work exclusively with the more challenging group of people with long-term mental distress and multiple problems. Case management has come into being precisely because this client group tended to be under-provided with services from all the traditional professions. The intensity of work, with small case-loads, should also distinguish this style of working from that generally performed by uni-professional teams.

There is a case, in the new teams, for brokering the injection and sectioning to specialist services. This is particularly important when we consider the greater significance given to the client–worker relationship. There is a vital need for each team member to feel a greater equality of responsibility, despite the different professional backgrounds, the statutory responsibilities which may be assumed by some professions can artificially skew the relationship between different team members and can certainly affect the quality of the client–worker relationship. However, logic does not always prevail, and these tend often to be very delicate local management issues when a new community multi-disciplinary team is to be established along principles of case management.

FURTHER TRAINING OR A NEW PROFESSION?

Much of the current debate in the UK is focused on training needs in order to develop a fully competent case manager, capable of providing the type of new service which may better meet the wants and needs of the clients experiencing long-term mental health problems who have a complexity of problems and difficulties in most aspects of their daily living. There is a very real danger of this debate polarizing between, on the one hand, existing professions insisting that their training is adequate to meet the needs of a fully functioning community service and, on the other hand, a mix of radical workers (professional and non-professional) stating the roles have very definite training needs which no single existing professional syllabus can satisfy. Research and Development for Psychiatry (RDP) are currently using their own researched national case management project to attempt to identify some of the specific training needs that workers from different backgrounds require in order to fulfil the remit of the new posts.

The longer experience of the US programmes has resulted in a more clearly defined identity for case managers, but more specific conclusions regarding training needs or professional status have still not been achieved. Kanter (1989) lists the need for trained clinical skills in assessment, treatment and service planning, consultation, supportive psychotherapy and crisis intervention. He suggests that no single profession includes such a comprehensive package in its training, but identifies specific professionals and non-professionals targeting gaps in their skills to dictate postgraduate training requirements. Witheridge (1989) broadens the debate by suggesting that 'certain aspects of the assertive community treatment worker's role cannot readily be taught. Because of their aptitudes, their interests, and even their temperaments, certain individuals are unquestionably cut out for the job: others are not. Furthermore, the correlation between suitability and prior professional training is weaker than one might expect it to be'. He identifies a revised training syllabus as needing to address:

- professional attitudes, values and beliefs;
- biological, psychological and sociological foundations;
- historical foundations of mental health professions;
- methods of intervention;

but still concludes with a need to abandon the narrow ideologies of traditional practice in order to 'experiment with innovative techniques whose merit has yet to be conclusively demonstrated'.

So the debate is still far from being conclusive, with the current emphasis still focusing on the more conservative approach of encouraging individuals to build on their initial professional training and using postgraduate opportunities to fill gaps. The position of the unqualified but highly experienced remains an under-used resource with significantly less status and pay. This ultimately represents a loss to the client group. Some programmes in the US have attempted to adopt a rational use of staff resources by employing lesser qualified people in the posts of case managers under the close supervision of more qualified pesonnel (Rapp and Wintersteen, 1989). The mix needs to be carefully addressed, particularly as clients will often respond differently to unqualified staff, perceiving their loyalties to be less entrenched in the system and consequently opening up in a different way on occasions.

STAFF SUPPORT

Staff support in community multi-disciplinary teams should not be seen as an isolated component but rather in conjunction with training, monitoring and management of the service (Pilling, 1991). Shepherd (1988b) highlights that within the specific client group there is still a hard core of untreatable disability (in the medical sense) requiring special skills to cope with potentially frustrating maintenance work. He suggests that the nature of the work demands people who remain optimistic whilst still being realistic about the potential outcome of interventions, and also that we need to investigate further what factors may influence staff morale, enthusiasm and effectiveness in these situations.

When addressing the specific work outlined in this chapter, we need to consider the types of support and management required to promote cohesive team development as well as the more obvious requirement for support and supervision for the individual worker. Onyett (1992) suggests that we need to address the issues of 'structure' and 'process' if we are to understand how teams can be successfully brought together. One of the first considerations of team structure should be the relationship of team management to each individual in the multi-disciplinary team. Onyett (1992) discusses roles for professional line managers or co-ordinators which give rise to the alternatives of the profession-managed network, the fully managed team or options for a co-ordinated team with shared management. Each carries its own advantages and disadvantages, but we must not ignore the final influence of the personalities of individuals, at management and team worker level, in determining the successful development of a multi-disciplinary team.

Patmore and Weaver (1991) suggest that multi-disciplinary teams are not unpredictable entities that simply 'gel together' through luck: they require consistency of planning and management. Watts and Bennett's (1991) study of the management of staff in multi-disciplinary teams recalls that hierarchical arrangements satisfy the circumstances where the likely problems are predictable, but more intricate networks of support and control are required for teams attempting innovative working methods where the problems tend to be more unpredictable. Furthermore, more flexible interaction between staff helps to reduce any potential resistance to innovation.

For the individual worker, good quality supervision should be an essential characteristic of team functioning from the outset, not just as a response after problems have arisen. A number of issues may need to be addressed when working in these situations:

- coping with difficult and demanding work, particularly where the pace of change is slow and there may be increased levels of client dependence;
- feeling a lack of technical skills to deal with all the demands of potentially challenging behaviours;
- innovative styles of work which go beyond the limits of the professional training;
- managing a sense of individual professional isolation, which may be accompanied by ambiguity over roles and professional identity;
- addressing personal and professional growth and development.

The price of inadequate or poorly planned support and supervision can be 'burn-out', characterized by apathy towards the context of the work and questioning one's own abilities. Hawkins and Shohet (1989) suggest 'burnout is not an illness that you catch, neither is it a recognisable event or state, for it is a process that often begins very early in one's career as a helper. Indeed its needs may be inherent in the belief systems of many of the helping professions and in the personalities of those who are attracted to them.' They suggest that one preventative approach is to ensure an adequate 'learning environment' is maintained throughout a career.

Formal arrangements for support

Supervision

This assumes the format of individual supervision with a line manager, but Hawkins and Shohet (1989) also outline a full discussion of self, group, team and peer supervision methods. In addition to addressing the issues outlined above, the activity should focus on case-load management, wider networking and service development issues, and team structure and cohesion.

Appraisals

These are likely to occur less often than supervision meetings; usually on a regular basis, for example, every six months. Appraisal is often used as a method of formally documenting personal and professional development through the mutual agreement of setting achievable objectives – agreed between the worker and line manager and monitored together at the next formal appraisal meeting. It is important that the objectives be designed to stretch the abilities of the individual worker, and they should range across all the functions associated with the post. The successful use of appraisal arises from selling it as an aid to promoting further development, not as a penalty for failure or as a method simply for checking up on a worker.

Line and professional management

By definition, the team leader of a multi-disciplinary team will not hold the same professional background as all the team members. In circumstances where individual workers may possibly experience ambiguity about their isolated or changing role, it is vital that provision be made for access to professional management, if required. However, we should be equally aware of the potential difficulties if a professional

manager disagrees with the developing philosophy of a
multi-disciplinary team and brings pressure to bear on their
professional representative(s) in the team. Equally destructive
consequences may result.

Job descriptions

Witheridge (1989) indicates the difficulty of being too specific
when writing a job description for a new and innovative post.
Where there is some disagreement between managers over
the style or method of working, or where there is a plan for
interchangeable roles, the individual worker should be offered
some protection and direction through the job description.
Benefits may accrue also from engaging individual workers
in periodic reviews of their job descriptions in line with the
periodic appraisals.

Operational policies

Patmore and Weaver (1991) suggest that their study of operational policies rarely showed them to present convincing
proposals for the day-to-day practice of multi-disciplinary
teamwork. They recommend that the client recruitment,
allocation and care planning policies should be planned well
in advance. I would also suggest that in the case of newly
developing teams a sense of ownership may be engendered
in team members if they are all encouraged to contribute to
the development of the operational policies and subsequent
reviews. Onyett (1992) outlines the main functions of an
operational policy and argues that it is only of real use if it
is 'part of an on-going service review process and should be
amenable to continuous revision'.

Team planning days

In addition to the regular team 'business' meetings, the whole
team can be encouraged to focus on its particular tasks and
desire for innovation if it can manage to take occasional 'time
out' to review its working methods and operational policies.
Time away from the day-to-day operational demands may also
allow the freedom of thought necessary to generate and consider new ideas.

management and the care programme also focus the attention on this administrative response (Ryan, Ford and Clifford, 1991).

The clinical model (Kanter, 1989) and the strengths model (Rapp and Wintersteen, 1989) of case management focus the attention more on an interactional response for team practice, whereby the core function becomes the individual client–case manager relationship upon which can be built the intensive and wide ranging forms of support. The client becomes the central focus and director of the helping process. If the various professions were to restrict themselves to core functions, much of the most important work of the multi-disciplinary teams would go undone. It would fail to make the best use of the staff, as most members of the team have skills that go beyond their professional core functions (Meteyard, 1990).

The successful functioning of the multi disciplinary team must be built on good networks of staff support (Watts and Bennett, 1991). This should be clearly integrated with the management and monitoring functions of the team from its inception (Pilling, 1991). Adequate support should address the issues of team cohesion and development as well as the supervision of the individual workers (Hawkins and Shohet, 1989).

3

Working methods: from theory into practice

One of the cornerstones of the development of any profession is its ability to refer to the theoretical frameworks which guide its practice. Though we may all wish to uphold our primary role as that of practitioner – with the emphasis on 'hands on practice' – we still need to acknowledge our place within a much larger system. We are required to offer our practice to numerous people, and we need to communicate and co-ordinate our actions as one among many professions and agencies.

We may only be respected, in a professional sense, when we are able to communicate the aims of our practice, the process we follow to achieve those aims and the basis for our beliefs in our own practice. Theories, models and frames of reference have been developed to provide the underlying rules which guide our practice and help us focus our interpretations of the information we receive.

Health care professions owe their theoretical development, in varying degrees, to four psychological approaches – analytical, behaviourial, humanistic and developmental. The growth of the occupational therapy profession has seen these theories give rise to a number of different models for practice, including:

- Cronin Mosey, adaptive skills;
- Llorens, facilitating growth and development;
- Reilly, occupational behaviour;
- Kielhofner, human occupation.

important that a worker should acknowledge what is being said and work with the content rather than make instant negative responses. Many clients have been all too familiar with negative reactions towards themselves or their ideas. They may also be testing you out by setting up an unreal situation to see how differently you may react from their usual experience of negative responses. A further note of caution on this point is the danger of colluding with a person's symptomatic fantasy world – once again, it is important not to belittle such ideas instantly, but to acknowledge the content and try to discuss its relation to reality as you perceive it to be. I have personally spent a substantial amount of time sitting on a chair in a bedroom while the resident remained hidden beneath the bedsheets, only for the person to finally emerge to discuss the qualities of dust in Morocco. After a number of visits following this routine we did manage to progress to more immediately relevant subjects for discussion centred around making plans for the future. Ultimately these situations require the skills of mental state assessment and active listening in a non-threatening manner.

4. Address more immediate practical issues. The focus of attention on one isolated practical issue that has the potential to be resolved can pay dividends in progressing engagement. Nothing breeds success quite like success. In its simplest form this may involve obtaining information about a resource, an outstanding appointment or a specific type of medication; it could involve setting up a new appointment or, in a more ambitious form, it may address a financial issue – a benefit entitlement, arrears, debts, a contested statement of account. The short history of the 'Poll Tax' in the UK may have caused untold confusion and disharmony across the country, but it has presented a golden opportunity for progressing engagement issues – particularly where you can achieve an agreement with the authorities to reduce an original demand of £300 down to £60, or even achieve total exemption.

5. Use humour. This can have a powerful effect, particularly for people whose lives may have been dominated by negative feelings with little opportunity to experience

light-hearted interactions. A word of caution is needed, however, because styles of humour can be misinterpreted, and ideally it should be used later in a meeting after assessing reactions to other forms of interaction. Do not walk straight in presenting your favourite comedy routine!

6. Maintain regular indirect contacts. Where possible an occasional telephone call, written letter, or a brief note through the letter box when you fail to gain an answer can prove effective in progressing a relationship. It can give the message that the person is not forgotten and that we aim to fulfil a promise to be around for them on a regular, long-term basis.

7. Continue with a minimum level of contact. This partially reflects a notion of client empowerment through less need for contact, but refers more to the situation where the person only permits occasional access, or only discusses a limited range of issues, but still does not actively request that you discontinue all contact. By continuing at the pace and to the agenda set by the client you may continue to indicate your interest in their welfare and fulfil any suggestions you may have made about responding to their directives.

My colleagues and I have built up experience of literally talking through closed doors when a client has wished to maintain only a tenuous link with the service. You also begin to develop an awareness of subtle indications of when a person is at home but not prepared to communicate with you – sounds of movement inside, patterns of opening or closing curtains or internal doors that signify whether a person is at home or not. Generally, they respond on the occasions most suited to them.

8. Worker self-disclosure. Guidelines about the giving of personal information to clients are generally loose and open to personal interpretation. This can be a potentially very powerful tool for engagement, because most clients are not accustomed to a two-way information giving relationship. Caution and discretion need to be applied in all cases. It is recommended that the worker should always question if any specific disclosures are to the benefit of relationship building, i.e. to the clients' ultimate benefit, and not as a personal release for the worker.

Graduated disengagement or discharge?

Within the strengths model the notion of graduated disengage-ment has developed to denote a tapering-off of direct contacts between a client and a case manager. Usually this should represent a situation where a client reaches a level of confi-dent functioning and no longer feels the desire for such intensive support but where they are still aware of the availability of someone they can contact to discuss progress or any subsequent issues that arise.

The concept of discharge has a sense of finality and termina-tion which is less relevant for a person being offered a service for life. It also tends to be a concept employed by services rather than by service users. There may, however, be occasional circumstances where discharge is indicated, for example, when a client moves out of a service catchment area or if the client is quite realistically adamant about not wanting contact with the service. Where possible, even in these situations, the process of discharge should be eased through, rather than be presented as a sudden and immediate event.

Circumstances where a client does not seem realistic about the desire for discharge need to be handled with equal care. This conclusion may just be a value judgement on the part of service providers who find difficulty 'letting go', but it needs to be explored from the point of view of a whole range of consequences for the individual concerned. The client should always be offered information for re-entry to services in the future, rather than being left with no prospect of options for advice and support.

ASSESSMENT

The government White Paper *Caring for People* (DOH, 1989) states that

> the aim of assessment should be to arrive at a decision on whether services should be provided, and in what form. Assessment will therefore have to be made against a background of stated objectives and priorities. Decisions on service provision will have to take account of what is available and affordable. Priority must be given to those whose needs are greatest.

Essentially, this statement seems to be more relevant to the managerial level of assessing what resources can be allocated to different service areas. Certainly, any practitioner would state that the clients experiencing severe distress are a high priority, since they will have experienced multiple needs over long periods of time with arguably insufficient and irrelevant resources allocated to them. Whether or not an individual is to receive a particular service is a function performed early on at the referral stage, set against the identified criteria for that service. True individual assessment begins after this decision has been made.

A problem-solving approach

Within the occupational therapy process assessment is seen as the first stage, with the purpose of gathering information about a person and his or her personal circumstances. The occupational therapist is seen as a 'problem-solver' who contributes specific assessment information to the total picture built up by a treatment team by focusing the assessment on clarifying functional problems regarding the person's life roles. Within these limits, Finlay (1988) suggests that clear assessment procedures are important for the occupational therapist to:

- understand the problem(s);
- recognize the individual needs;
- identify the baseline for treatment; and
- evaluate future progress.

Whilst the focus is problem-orientated, occupational therapists also tend to highlight a need to discover the individual's strengths and abilities, both in order to complete an assessment of the personal situation and to anchor treatment to positive attributes where possible. In this respect, Willson (1987) suggests that a complete view of a person's situation is only made possible by also addressing:

- attributes and attitudes;
- barriers and battles;
- capabilities and choices.

Strengths assessment approach

Rapp (1988) suggests that the typical assessment processes practised by mental health professionals can have a depressing effect on the individual's motivation, simply through their emphasis on the negative aspects of personal circumstances. He suggests that 'work with clients should not be directed at their symtomatology, psychosis or, for that matter, problems, weaknesses and deficits. Rather the work should focus on what the client has done, what resources have been or are currently available to the client, what the client knows, and what aspirations and dreams they may hold.'

The purpose of a strengths assessment across all aspects of the person's life should not be the building of a list of 'needs' as perceived by the worker but a statement of wants as perceived by the client. This should guide the direction of personal and social resources towards accomplishing what is desired (Rapp and Kisthardt, 1991; Weick 1989). The guidelines for conducting a strengths assessment outlined below are developed from the work of Rapp and Kisthardt (1991).

To be useful as a tool in the case management helping process, the strengths assessment should be:

- focused on the gathering of information in the main areas of needs and wants relative to each individual's current circumstances; what, if anything, they wish to achieve or acquire in each area and what involvements or resources they have used in the past in each area;
- ongoing; circumstances and desires change, assessment is not static and absolute and new facts of a person continuously emerge;
- conducted in a conversational manner, not a structured interview;
- developed at each individual's own pace and comfort level;
- as detailed and specific as possible and should clearly individualize each person;
- useful in partializing the many areas of a person's life in which they have wants and needs;
- hopeful, uplifting and even a fun process for individual clients and case managers;

Table 3.1 Case management: consumer strengths assessment

Case Manager's Name: S. Morgan	Consumer's Name: Mrs F.	Date: 29/10/91
Current status *What's going on today?* *What's available now?*	*Individual's desires/* *aspirations: What do I want?*	*Resources, personal/* *social: What have I used in the* *past?*
	Life domain	
	Daily living situation	
Lives in one-bedroomed well-maintained council flat. Enjoys cooking.	Wishes to regain care of her daughter.	Settled in tenancy for one year. Cared for daughter for six years.
	Financial/insurance	
Receives Income Support and Housing Benefit.	Wishes to increase income without pressures of full-time work.	Held a number of short-term, part-time cleaning jobs.
	Vocational/educational	
Currently unemployed. Attends drop-in centre 1 ×/week.	Return to part-time employment within own tolerance of stress.	(See Financial) Enjoys getting on with individual tasks.
	Social supports	
Drop-in centre visits. Case Manager visits. No contact with family.	12-year old daughter to return home from foster care.	Family together for few years. One-year stay in women's hostel.

Health

Feeling not too stressed. Wrists still painful from past fractures.	Monitor own stress to remain out of hospital.	Reduce levels of activity if feeling stressed and lethargic.

Leisure/recreational supports

Watches soap operas and horse racing on TV.	Wishes to share more time with her daughter.	Watching television. Relaxation. Contacts at day centres.

What are my priorities?

1. 'The return of my daughter;'
2. 'to keep my flat;'
3. 'to return to part-time work;'
4. 'no more admissions to hospital.'

Case Manager's comments:
'Mrs F. is now more certain about her own wishes'.

Consumer's comments:
'I feel more settled in my own flat'.

Case manager's signature:	Date:	Consumer's signature:	Date:
S. Morgan	4.11.91	Mrs F.	4.11.91

(Source: Rapp and Kisthardt, 1991; published with kind permission.)

- paint a holistic portrait of each client's life; strengths noted in one area may be useful in promoting successful goal attainment in another area;
- clearly and logically related to the specific helping plans that are recorded on the personal plan.

In a strengths approach the 'needs' are not ignored but should be channelled towards the achievement of the 'wants'. So, if a person wants to be an occupational therapist but has difficulty getting out of bed in the morning and lacks the motivation to attend to personal appearance and hygiene the problem-solving approach would target the problem areas and devise a programme of activity to challenge the problem behaviours; a strengths approach would focus attention on the desired goal of being an occupational therapist and discuss what behaviours may be needed to achieve the goal. The difference is one of positive and negative focus (see Table 3.1 for an example of a written Strengths Assessment). It is likely that the client generally regarded to be unmotivated is more likely to respond to a positive focus than to a negative focus which highlights the problems.

Location of assessment

Many occupational therapists stress the importance of their 'department' as a valuable resource for assessment, particularly if it is adequately stocked with materials and equipment. Some occupational therapists, through personal philosophy or location of their work in the community, stress the vital importance of assessment in the home rather than in simulated environments. Both have their value across the generic range of the work undertaken by occupational therapy as a profession but, in the case of the specific client group with long-term difficulties, the simulated environment has more limited advantages. Ultimately, assessment should be about the interaction of individuals and their environment – they will behave differently in different situations and will not necessarily translate skills from one to another location. Pilling (1991) explores many of the issues of hospital-based rehabilitation programmes, but also indicates that hospital-based assessment for community resettlement purposes is a poor prediction of future success in the community.

Time-scales for assessment

This is one aspect of the process which enjoys a wide-ranging consensus view – assessment should not be seen as a stage to be completed before moving on to the next stage of the process. While the term 'initial assessment' may be used to denote the early stages of gathering basic information through gradual engagement, it is seen as an ongoing requirement which constantly takes account of changing situations, wants, values and needs. It should be guided by a framework which allows and encourages the client to be the central part of the procedure.

Methods of assessment

A number of references give an introduction to formal methods of assessment: observation, interviews, self-rating scales, standardized tests, performance checks (Willson, 1987; Finlay, 1988; Creek, 1990). Rapp and Kisthardt (1991) remind us of the vital importance of the continuing assessment in informal settings: at home, in the café, park, place of work. Some clients clearly illustrate the principles of behaviour theories by exhibiting learned behaviour when they enter a clinical setting then assuming their more natural behaviours when away from the clinical setting.

A distinction can also be made between quantitative and qualitative methods of assessment. The former are essentially outcome evaluations concerned with value for money. Qualitative methods are more specific to our concerns here, addressing the detailed analysis of a person's strengths and difficulties, wants and needs (Meteyard, 1990; Shepherd, 1988a). But any particular team will tend to adopt the assessment method which best suits the situation it finds itself in.

CARE PLANNING

The essential function of this aspect of the process is to bring together and collate all the information that has been collected through engagement and assessment in order to reach an agreement on what is wanted and needed and to draw up some priorities for action in the form of goals and objectives (Pilling, 1991).

There again appears to be some considerable agreement, in theory, on how to present a goal or objective. In general, a statement of goals and objectives should be:

- practically obtainable;
- measurable;
- established in agreement with the client;
- acknowledging resource or environmental constraints;
- reviewed at agreed intervals.

Rapp (1988) concludes from his examination of many examples of care plans that practitioners across all services have fallen into the bad practice of writing a very limited range of generalized goals, such as:

- improve personal appearance
- improve daily living skills
- improve socialization skills
- improve prevocational skills
- take medication as prescribed
- attend appointments and follow treatment plan.

He concludes that not only is this bad practice but it portrays the clients as an homogeneous group with no reflection of individual character and circumstances.

A problem-solving approach

The occupational therapist will draw up a personal specific treatment plan to be co-ordinated with the plans of other professions. The focus is still that of organizing information to identify and prioritize problem areas to be tackled and may, secondarily, identify strengths and abilities that can be utilized in the treatment of these problems. Within the priorities, emphasis is placed on separating out short, medium and long-term goals. The care plan or treatment plan will also specify the selected activity and personal and environmental factors that may influence the outcomes.

A strengths model approach

Much more emphasis is placed on a case manager supporting clients to select their own goals, always in the form of short-term achievable goals. This function often shares the occupational therapy core skill of activity analysis by encouraging the client to break down an activity into its component parts so that the goals can be made more specific to achieving success in small compartmentalized areas, leading to overall achievement in larger aspects of what is desired.

The goal-planning process is guided by a belief that people grow by building on successful activities in areas of their lives that hold more personal meaning. Small successes are expected to breed further success by concentrating on the skills the client feels most capable in. The client is encouraged to keep duplicate copies of the care planning documents and to periodically review and update them with the case manager. Such a process should be flexible enough to progress at the pace set by the individual client. (An example of a 'Case Management Personal Plan' is in Table 3.2.)

EVALUATION

This function is often considered to be, theoretically, the final part of the occupational therapy process, though the fluid nature of the whole process necessarily means it leads on to a modification of our practice as we continually reassess the situation and alter the goals and priorities for work with the client.

The concept of 'evaluation' covers similar functions at three different levels:

1. reviewing progress with an individual client;
2. formal reporting of outcome results;
3. wider research into a complete service.

Shepherd (1988a) suggests that the process of monitoring and evaluating services has become increasingly important in recent years, because both the public and politicians are demanding much greater accountability for the various agencies providing care.

Table 3.2 Case management personal plan

For: Mrs F. Case Manager: S. MORGAN Date: 18.11.91

Planned frequency of contact: 1×/week

Life domain focused upon:

—	Daily living situation
×	Social supports
—	Financial/insurance
—	Vocational/educational
—	Leisure/recreational supports
—	Health

Measurable short-term goals toward achievement	Responsibility	Date to be accomplished	Date accomplished	Comments
1. Mrs F. Will accept a home visit by her daughter's social worker.	Mrs F. and S. Morgan	18.11.91	18.11.91	Mrs F. offered a cup of tea to SW to begin the meeting.
2. Mrs F. will use at least 15 mins of each meeting with CM to discuss feelings about her child being in care.	Mrs F. and S Morgan	17.12.91	17.12.91	After the first meeting Mrs F. was able to discuss her feelings.
3. Mrs F. will commence weekly supervised meetings with daughter in the Social Services office.	Mrs F.	10.12.91	10.12.91	Mrs F. coped well with a very emotional reunion, 6 years apart.
4. Mrs F. will use CM meetings to discuss her daughter's progress.	Mrs F. and S. Morgan	17.12.91	17.12.91	Expressing positive feelings about her daughter's social and academic progress.

Consumer's signature: Date:
Mrs F.   18.11.91
Dr P.   20.11.91

Case Manager's signature: Date:
S. Morgan   18.11.91
_____   _____

(Source: Rapp and Kisthardt, 1991; published with kind permission.)

In this chapter we are more concerned with the level of individual client reviews, a process that Rapp and Kisthardt (1991) refer to as 'collective and continuous collaboration'. Once again, the individual client should be seen as the central figure, but all involved agencies should collaborate to assist the client to sustain the achievements gained.

Pilling (1991) suggests that the function of evaluation can be a threatening and anxiety-provoking experience for both the clients and the professionals involved. Particularly with this client group, the pace of change can be extremely slow and difficult to achieve. In this sense, evaluation may be seen as a method of highlighting failings, though it can also be the catalyst for highlighting the successes, which may not be as visible as in other areas of work.

Who undertakes the evaluation

Essentially, the client should be involved in all aspects of discussing progress and monitoring changes to priorities and goals. The particular case manager will initiate the formal or informal discussions, but it is also the workers' role to undertake the administration of paperwork. Reviews will ideally involve all the personnel directly concerned in the delivery of services to the individual.

When should evaluation take place?

Informal discussions between client and worker or worker and worker will be an ongoing function, much the same as the assessment. Formal reviews should have an agreed timetable and location to best ensure the fullest possible contribution of all relevant people. Three to six months is the most common frequency for such reviews, and the case manager should undertake the responsibility to co-ordinate the necessary arrangements to ensure it takes place.

Reviews within specific team meetings would be organized within the protocol set by the team. They may or may not invite the client or outside workers into such a meeting. In the event of the client not being involved, such a review should take the form of team supervision rather than a formal client review.

There may be circumstances in which the client expresses no wish to be involved in the 'bureaucracy' of organizational functioning.

Where can evaluation take place?

The location is variable, depending on client preference, who is to be involved and what specific purposes the evaluation is to address. Review meetings in clinical settings – office, ward, department will usually follow a loosely defined protocol common to the management of organizations. This may include the formalities of minutes, chairperson, agendas and formal invitations to attend.

Reviews in community-based services are frequently held in a wide variety of settings – the client's home, centre for day care, office base, park bench, café. There may often be a greater degree of informality more suited to the clients themselves; but the more public the location, the more crucial it is to attend to all aspects of confidentiality.

In my own experience, there have been occasions when a small group of workers arrived at a client's flat for the purpose of review only to find that the client gets up and walks out of the flat in the middle of the meeting, leaving the workers to continue the meeting in the client's home but without the most significant person. The prime lesson was to address tolerance for sitting through the unnatural situation of a formalized meeting, even in an informal environment.

SUMMARY

Occupational therapy shares with the other professions a process which helps us to rationalize, organize, document and communicate the work we undertake in practice (Finlay, 1988). Although there is general agreement on the main elements, first to communicate with the client, leading on to assessing, planning and evaluating our interactions, the models for the approach differ in their underlying principles.

The generic mental health professions adopt an outlook that stresses the importance of assessment as the first function in their process (Willson, 1987; Finlay, 1988). The Personal Strengths Model of Case Management contrasts with this situation; firstly, by specifying a more narrowly defined client group, and, secondly, in its belief that engagement is the vital first element upon which all subsequent functions of the process can be built (Rapp and Kisthardt, 1991).

The 'problems' and 'strengths' approaches contrast on other significant issues of philosophy. Problems are finite and common; they are shared by us all but experienced in an individualized and personal way. Our strengths tend to be much more idiosyncratic and more clearly express our individuality (Rapp, 1988). Ultimately, people progress and grow through building on their abilities and diversifying their interests. A focus on defining problems can only serve to highlight liabilities, which is a far more difficult starting point from which to launch positive change.

4

Medical and psychosocial
interventions

The client group for whom we are particularly concerned have
been identified in the introductory chapter, but in order to set
the medical context refer to Wing and Morris (1981) who state:

> The commonest psychiatric diagnosis among people who
> use high dependency services is schizophrenia, but manic-
> depressive disorders, severe and chronic neurosis, and
> personality disorders are also frequent. . . . Moreover, many
> people have multiple impairments; the diagnosis of psychi-
> atric disorder is associated with physical disability, blind-
> ness, deafness, epilepsy, alcohol or drug abuse.

They further suggest that detailed knowledge of the specific
impairments of each individual is essential if rehabilitation is
to be tailored to personal need. In general terms, the com-
monest syndrome of chronic schizophrenia is 'social withdrawal, flatness of affect, slowness, underactivity, poverty of
speech, apathy, self-neglect, difficulty in using non-verbal as
well as verbal communication – the so-called 'negative
symptoms'.

The focus of this chapter will not be the theoretical
understanding of psychiatric symptomatology; such discussions are widely published in general psychiatry texts (Hughes,
1990; Goldman, 1988). I am more concerned here with the
manifestation of psychiatric impairments in the community
and the types of medical and psychosocial support required
and offered as a response to the experiences of mental distress.
Shepherd (1991) states that '''chronic'' patients, by definition,

suffer with persistent and sometimes intractable symptoms and for them the goal of symptom relief is often not realistic. Instead, one has to try to help them develop their functional abilities and, at the very least, enable them to function at an optimal level despite their symptoms. "Symptoms" and "functioning" must therefore be considered as potentially independent domains.' Realistically, we are looking to support a person's ability to 'manage and cope with the experience of distress', rather than the more ideological standpoint of 'treating and curing an illness'.

In this chapter, I am also concerned about the continuing relationship between the hospital and the community. Much of the debate has tended to unnecessarily polarize into an either/or response, once again denying the individuality of the person by assuming that one type of solution will suit all. Despite the undeniable vagaries of an institutional system, there are still many clients who feel a sense of security and reassurance from knowing that the hospital will be there in their times of greatest distress. Not all hospital units should be seen as offering poor and degrading services; the focus of the service has changed significantly since the 1950s and the prime aim should now be to offer choices to the clients that they feel could best meet their needs. The concept of choice should particularly extend to the notions of 'asylum' or 'retreat', so a range of options should be available to meet the different perceptions of what feels safe and secure at times of severe distress.

The changing emphasis from institutional care to community care brings with it a need for the medical model to change from its more diagnostic and prescriptive emphasis and adapt to the influences of different environmental circumstances to become more flexible in the face of client wants. Very subtle shifts of power accompany the delivery of services on the client's home ground. Whilst the power differential still lies appreciably in favour of the professionals, doctors no longer have that extra air of authority that is conferred by white coats and offices at the end of long corridors. Furthermore, the psychiatrist is no longer the whole arbiter of medical services. In the community setting, the GP adopts a much higher profile in service provision than when the focus of attention was internalized in the institution.

Many of the positive changes that are recently altering the delivery of psychiatric services are a direct consequence of the greater collaboration between people, professional or non-professional, medical or non-medical. The shifts of power that occur with a focus in the community have provided a strong incentive for addressing the importance of good communication between all relevant people.

Medication still remains largely the treatment of choice for chronic mental health problems, though the desire for such a standpoint is greatly questioned from many sources, not the least of which are the recipients themselves. Although there is a strong focus on the medication issues in this chapter, I do not wish to imply this is the only form of treatment offered. Much work has developed around a number of concepts such as life events, high expressed emotion and other psychosocial interventions.

It has been my intention, however, to separate out that which is more usually seen as 'medical care' from the medical involvement in the various aspects of psychosocial interventions. To this end I will be concentrating on the medical relationships of hospital and community, the manifestation of distress seen in the community (using the profile and case material), the psychiatrist and GP relationship, the need for greater liaison and networking and the more controversial issues of medication and compulsory detention. Additionally, I will make brief references to some of the more recent psychosocial developments.

THE RELATIONSHIP OF HOSPITAL TO COMMUNITY

The historical development of the hospital closure programme, or 'deinstitutionalization', with the simultaneous emphasis on providing mental health services under the umbrella term of 'community care' has been well charted (Ramon, 1988; Watts and Bennett, 1991). But there has been the very real pitfall of looking to the two extreme ends of the spectrum, in an 'all or nothing' attitude towards the shifting pattern of service provision. This polarization of the debate into a question of whether care should be provided in the hospital or in the community is the result of professional debates that tend to exclude the all-important voice of the service user. Nor are these views necessarily based on sound research foundations.

Wing and Morris (1981) summarized the two sides of the debate as being the fear of a swing back to the custodial era (as long as the institutions remained intact) against the fear of the inevitable difficulties that will arise for the afflicted person, the relatives and society in general if we deny real disability by adopting unrealistic expectations. The polarity of views also appears to be fuelled by the notion that the growth of community care will be financed by the hospital closure programme. The reality of the early 1990s appears to be that of mental hospitals continuing to close: community services are growing in a somewhat uneven and haphazard manner and users, relatives and many professionals fear for the future ability of services to meet needs. Certainly current provision of community services does not seem to match the information we are receiving about levels of need.

More realistically, Pilling (1991) argues that community care will not be achieved by only moving resources from the hospital site to a variety of community sites. Hospital care should continue to be 'a key component of any community-based service'. Despite the continual decrease in the numbers of people in long-stay hospital beds for the foreseeable future, people with long-term mental health problems may require shorter periods of in-patient admission (many by their own choice) due to the exacerbation of severe distress.

Following this line of argument, the psychiatric in-patient unit should be seen as a community resource in its own right, serving the community needs of its geographical catchment area. Pilling (1991) suggests that we should not emphasize 'the primacy of the hospital in community care, but rather that hospital care has an important role to play in the provision of community mental health services'.

We should now restructure the debate from the fixed views of the mental hospital service or community to an investigation of what type of hospital services will continue to be necessary to meet specific community needs. The smaller psychiatric hospitals located within their local communities may well continue to have a valuable contribution to offer as a community service. These need to be evaluated alongside the options of smaller psychiatric units in District General

Hospitals and the more recent development of smaller hostel-wards which can provide intensive nursing care 24 hours a day for groups of up to 20 residents and link into the local health services of the area.

Wing and Morris (1981) have suggested that the psychiatric units of the District General Hospital are not very conducive to the rehabilitation of the long-stay patient because of the clinical atmosphere and philosophy of rapid turnover of bed usage. In the case of the hostel-wards, the criticisms tend to focus on their potential to replicate the institutional nature of the larger hospitals; but they do provide the possibility of a permanent home in the local community for those few people who, for whatever reasons, are incapable of independent living and need more support than relatives and other domiciliary services could offer. The hostel-ward also need not to become too institutional with properly trained staff.

For the majority of people who are able to achieve some degree of independent functioning in the community there is a need for a form of hospital care to operate within the overall community service. This is not an argument for keeping large mental hospitals open, but it does acknowledge a need to be clear about the purpose and function of some form of in-patient care for people who experience persistent severe mental distress. This need not be in a hospital structure, and it tends to link closely with the other debate over the question of 'asylum'.

THE NATURE OF ASYLUM

Historically, the term 'asylum' was a name given to the large old Victorian institution. It replaced the 'madhouse' label and became associated with 'lunatic' – the lunatic asylums. In this sense it is synonymous with the custodial era of management. It finally came to be replaced, in the 1930s, by 'mental hospital'.

More recently it has re-emerged with a more functional than descriptive meaning – J. Laurence (reported in Meteyard, 1990) suggests that asylum be defined as 'a safe place of refuge or shelter providing protection and support'. Many of the more traditional professionals and carers still link this to the old notion of the lunatic asylum, so they still consider there is a need for long-term accommodation of those people deemed incapable of independent living who would otherwise place an intolerable burden on their relatives.

The more radical professionals and groups representing service users, emphasize the distinction of choice when defining true asylum; it should be a place of refuge or sanctuary where a person chooses to go in periods of acute distress or exacerbation of long-term problems, and it should be made available for the period of time required by the individual. A distinction is made between the ability to choose asylum or being given care where the choice is denied.

As stated in the previous section, the place where asylum can be offered need not, some may say should not, be in a hospital setting. If we are clear about the purpose and function of what is being required and what is being offered, then the place of asylum could quite easily be on a more human scale, such as a 'safe house' in the community. Nevertheless there are likely to be occasions when acute exacerbations are in need of compulsory treatment, so any community provision should be able to encompass Mental Health Act patients.

MANIFESTATIONS OF MENTAL DISTRESS

The following profile and case material is presented at this point to build a picture of examples of real experiences of mental health difficulties as they present themselves for people living in the community.

PERSONAL PROFILE

Edwin is a 60-year-old man, of Jamaican origin, who has lived in the UK since 1957. He was married at the age of 57 to a 54-year-old widow with two daughters, one son and two grandsons from her previous marriage. Edwin has no regular contact with his own five siblings. They have shared a one-bedroom council flat on the second floor of a tower block since their marriage.

In medical terms, Edwin is diagnosed as suffering from chronic schizophrenia, having experienced persistent mental distress for 20 years, characterized by a strongly held and elaborately developed delusional system, focused around visual and tactile hallucinations. He makes constant reference to a conspiracy to persecute him, believing there to be collusion between M.I.5, M.I.6, police, hospital, Jamaican High Commission, the church and the local council. It is believed that they planted the neighbour in the flat above him with the specific purpose of pouring acid and hot dust through his ceiling on to him. At times, when his distress is more intense, he claims the dust drops on him wherever he is (indoors or outdoors) and no amount of logical discussion will move him from this fixed belief. He always wears a hat and will, on occasions, drape towels over his shoulders and balance a cushion or partly filled bowl of cold water on his head in the hope it will counteract his delusional beliefs. His wife will occasionally support his story with reference to her own experience of a burning sensation on her forearms whilst in bed, and sometimes attributes the experiences to supernatural phenomena. (She has no history of mental health problems.)

Edwin also occasionally refers to his belief that a worm lives within his body and that he has previously seen it surface under his arm. He doesn't relate this in any way to his other persecutory beliefs, but it has previously caused him to wear newspapers underneath his normal clothing.

Edwin has been admitted to psychiatric wards on six occasions, generally involuntarily, for periods ranging from two months up to one year. Large quantitites of oral and intramuscular neuroleptic medication have reduced his agitation and help reduce his preoccupation but has not relieved him of his delusional belief. Strong objections to the injections, by Edwin and his wife, on the grounds of intolerable weight gain and sexual impotence side-effects resulted in his refusal to continue taking them, but he continues to use oral medication comparatively frequently.

People who have known Edwin for a number of years indicate that the support and responsibilities within the marriage have had a more significant influence on calming his distress. His wife provides the basis of much stronger emotional support than he has previously known, and due to her physical disabilities (stroke, diabetes, hyper-tension) he is required to fulfil a greater responsibility for the practical tasks of daily living, which consequently help give him a structure to his time. Further structure is offered by his weekly attendance at two day centres – one a mental health resource, the other a club for elderly black people. A particular cause of frustration has been his inability to secure any meaningful paid employment since 1979.

The local council has previously accepted responsibility for rehousing Edwin on the grounds that he is vulner-able, representing a potential target for harassment on racial and mental health grounds. They have been aware that he complains of the same 'symptoms' in every tenancy that he has occupied. He is currently seeking a move from his tenancy on the grounds of the same per-secutory feelings, but also because his wife finds diffi-culty with mobility outside the flat – her friends and a potential day centre place are some miles away. The council is currently not giving the application a high priority because he is not being harassed in any way in his current location.

Edwin and his wife both receive invalidity benefit, in Edwin's name. They would be entitled to other benefits and rebates but generally experience great difficulty under-standing the social security system and completing the necessary application forms. Edwin has also built up large debts on the rent account by virtue of misunderstanding his entitlements and other people not being patient enough to try to understand his difficult speech and consequently not advising and helping him correctly.

To add to their difficulties, a daughter and grandson from his wife's previous marriage became homeless and have been using Edwin's living room as their home rather than accept the council's offer of bed and breakfast accom-modation. The pressures of overcrowding have been further compounded by the daughter taking advantage of the child-minding potential of Edwin and his wife and abusing the use of their telephone, leaving them with a further debt of over £800. The much needed phone is now on 'in-coming' calls only with the threat of disconnection if they do not meet a monthly repayment of £60.

Positive characteristics

- He has a strong, mutually supportive marital relationship which helps to highlight a warmth of personality in Edwin.
- He is comparatively satisfied with his daily routine of activity, though he would still prefer paid employment.
- He is very tolerant of people who have difficulty understanding his speech and ask him to repeat what he says.
- He consistently considers and verbalizes his need for help and support.

Needs identified by Edwin:

- the removal of the tenant upstairs whom he perceives to be the focus of the persecutory actions against him;
- help and advice with official information received through the post, e.g. bills, benefits and applications;
- a consistent and regular person to whom he can relate all his anxieties about the distress he experiences.

CASE STUDY 1

Losing the focus on reality

George is a 67-year-old man, born in England. His experience of severe mental distress originated in 1957 when he was 33 years of age and led on to what can only be referred to as a lifetime dominated by the controlling influence of experiences that appear very real to him but totally illogical to others who make contact with him. The result has been many years spent in long admissions to an old psychiatric institution with little change to the type of distress he experiences.

In medical terms, George has been diagnosed with chronic schizophrenia, following the consistent description of experiencing persistent auditory hallucinations, grandiose and persecutory delusions and passivity phenomena. These symptoms appear to be extremely pervasive, limiting his engagement in routines of daily activity to the very minimal, eating, drinking, sleeping and smoking.

He frequently believes himself to be the illegitimate off-spring of an Anglo-Russian royal affair and that he will ultimately receive five separate inheritances. He also believes himself to be a 'zombie' occupied by a woman who controls his every thought and movement. He constantly hears women's voices in his head, sometimes talking about him and sometimes to him. They are frequently persecutory, telling him he has killed people in the past, his food is poisoned and he is receiving someone else's medication. He also claims to frequently hear the screams of a dismembered body, tormented by any action he may make; as a result he believes that individual actions, e.g. smoking a cigarette or removing his coat, are wrong because they persecute somebody else. He also experiences a delusional idea that his tobacco and food is made up of 'spider's hormones'.

Regular medication over long periods of time has done little to resolve the distress George feels, and he tends to live a very socially isolated life, with the thoughts and the voices his only permanent companion. Dramatic changes have occurred for short periods of time following signifi-cant environmental change – shortly after moving to a smaller, more homely, hostel he appeared to completely recover overnight, denying any experience of symptoms, with full memory of his recent symptomatic experiences and remarkably retaining his personality that he recognized from 35 years previously. Sadly, his return to the same symptomatic condition was just as dramatic some two months later.

CASE STUDY 2

Medication compliance may present its own problems

Mary is a 56-year-old lady, profiled in more detail in the introduction. Her medical diagnosis of schizophrenia dates back some 36 years and her first psychiatric hospital admission lasted some 20 years. Persistent experiences of auditory hallucinations, self-neglect and social isolation are also compounded with severe physical disabilities and tremors, partly related to a thyroid problem and partly to long-term use of neuroleptic medication.

Mary frequently verbalizes the importance of taking medication to keep her well, but her extremely chaotic interpretation of instructions frequently results in her intake of more or less than the officially prescribed doses. The complex range of medication prescribed for physical and mental problems, and the inclusion of steroids, requires close monitoring of prescribed doses. Methods of enabling monitoring are discussed later in the chapter, but in Mary's case the use of a dosett box (described later) still results in her frequently taking a whole week's supply of medication in one day. She will attend surgeries for monthly injections if reminded of the time and date on the particular day; but Mary inevitably presents the potential problems of toxicity from unintentional overdosing on medication rather than the more common problems of people who refuse to take much of the medication prescribed.

THE PSYCHIATRIST AND THE GENERAL PRACTITIONER

The 1980s have seen increased activity in hospital closures, but up to this time the focus of attention for delivering services to people with persistent experiences of severe mental distress was the large mental hospital. The traditional medical model approach upheld the psychiatrist as the primary agent of care, where the distress was interpreted as being akin to other physical illnesses (though less well understood) requiring accurate diagnosis from which to plan largely physical treatment – medication, ECT, psychosurgery. Rehabilitation, in the sense of adopting functional skills to environmental circumstances, tended to take a more secondary role and remained limited to the simulated world of the hospital setting, very distant from the reality of the individual circumstances beyond the hospital gates. In fact, to some psychiatrists rehabilitation was, and still is, the product of successful physical treatments.

Many others have, however, become more fully aware of the social and environmental aspects of the experience of mental distress. Whilst many psychiatrists are actively supportive of an eclectic approach to treatments, the ability to implement a range of options is also partially determined by economics – hospital and medication still appearing to be the cheapest and most available solutions.

It was not until Shepherd *et al* (1981) reported their initial findings in 1966 that we began to acknowledge that most experiences of mental distress escape detection by the formal mental health services and that it is in fact the GP, not the psychiatrist, who assumes the larger responsibility for the care of people in distress. Furthermore, we must not jump to the rapid conclusion that the GP manages the less severe manifestations of distress and refers the more severe cases to the specialists: a more intensive sub-study of what was identified as '100 chronic psychiatric cases' revealed that only about one third of these people had ever been seen by a psychiatrist, and only six were in current contact with formal psychiatric services at the time of interview (Shepherd *et al.*, 1981).

The main reasons quoted for not referring those people on to psychiatrists were:

- the stigma associated with formal psychiatric care;
- a lowered opinion, by the GPs, of traditional psychiatric care being able to have any appreciable impact on severe disability;
- the inconsistent referral criteria adopted by psychiatrists.

The conclusions reached by Shepherd *et al.* clearly suggested that 'the cardinal requirements for the improvement of the mental health services in this country is not a large expansion and proliferation of psychiatric agencies, but rather a strengthening of the family doctor and his therapeutic role'.

However, the evidence also pointed to the continuing predominance of a medical approach. For people experiencing more severe episodes of distress, the GPs are more likely to see their function as focusing on diagnosis and the prescription of psychotropic medication than would be the case for the more specialist role of the psychiatrist.

As the concept of community care continues to advance, the GP's dominant role in managing severe mental distress strengthened. We are now witnessing a changing emphasis where psychiatrists are collaborating more effectively with the primary care medical services, providing specialist support services which help to re-enforce the GP's role as an effective member of the mental health team. It is equally necessary that other professional team members, in specialist psychiatric support services, should collaborate with the GP and psychiatrist in order to offer a wider view of the services that can be offered to the client who experiences severe distress manifesting itself in many different forms. The power base in psychiatric care is gradually shifting: there is an increasing acknowledgement of the experiences of 'real' problems occurring in the client's own community; the provision of a service requires more negotiation with the client, with rather less of the subtle coercive prescription to the client.

The medical model approach developed to reflect these changing circumstances is the biopsychosocial model, which is a more eclectic view attending to all facets of an individual's situation. Doctors have often been the pioneers of new social approaches, at the forefront of research into new developments and often actively supportive of innovative approaches deriving from multi-disciplinary collaboration.

The successful establishment of such collaboration derives from a common philosophy towards an area of working shared by people from many different backgrounds. It is built on respect for personal and professional skills, fostered through regular meetings and discussions and through taking opportunities to develop joint working practices. Time must always be found to communicate what is happening to all relevant people.

THE MONITORING OF MENTAL HEALTH

History-taking and present state examination

Technological advances in general medicine have contributed far less to the practice of psychiatry than to that of medicine and surgery, and the psychiatrist has to rely mainly on clinical observations through the medium of interpersonal communication. By far the most significant tool, in the tradition of psychiatry, is that of accurate diagnosis. Richter (1984) is representative of most of the literature in suggesting that the value of a diagnosis lies in its indications of the appropriate treatments and in guiding the psychiatrist to an idea of the prognosis for the disorder. Diagnosis is also an important starting point for understanding aetiology and developing new treatments.

In arriving at a diagnosis, the psychiatrist is entirely dependent on skill in taking a 'history' and an examination of the patient's mental state (and physical state, when indicated). Whilst a great deal of importance is attached to these procedures, it is also acknowledged that there may be differing opinions on their interpretation; such that 'disagreement amongst psychiatrists is not confined to diagnostic categories but also extends to the definition of symptoms. Again there is no way of externally validating symptoms, only a consensus of agreement'. (Leff and Isaccs, 1990.)

The procedures of history-taking and mental state examinations could have a much broader value to people other than psychiatrists who are involved in the support and management of mental distress. Although there is always the danger of stigmatized labelling through confirming a diagnosis, I would also suggest that these procedures, conducted in a non-threatening manner and environment, can help in other less medical ways. For the mental health professional, voluntary agency worker or user group representative, this approach of history-taking and assessment of mental state could be of some value in 'making contact' with a client, in establishing a useful rapport on which to build a working relationship, particularly if it is combined with the principles of a personal strengths approach as outlined in previous chapters.

I would again refer you to Leff and Isaccs (1990) for a readable account of how to conduct these procedures, but the following checklist can be committed to memory for practical reference:

1. Client History
   (a) History of present condition (including: starting point, development, severity and possible precipitant of distress).

(b) Personal background
- family history (including: ages, education, occupations, illnesses and any causes of death of parents and siblings);
- personal history (including: development milestones, occupational record, sexual orientation, social circumstances);
- previous history of physical, psychological or forensic problems;
- outline of personality when not experiencing severe distress.

2. Mental state examination
  (a) Non-verbal behaviour
  - dress
  - gait
  - motor activity
  - social manner and presentation
  - facial expressions.
  (b) Verbal behaviour
  - rate and quantity of speech
  - volume and tone of speech
  - non-social speech (i.e. talking to self)
  - speech disorders, reflecting disordered patterns of thought
  - neologisms (inventing new words)
  - changing topics
  - vagueness.
  (c) Psychiatric symptoms
  - delusions
  - hallucinations
  - signs of depression or anxiety
  - obsessions and phobias
  - suicidal thoughts or aggressive impulses.

When working in settings encountering acute or emergency episodes of distress, such as the psychiatric ward, psychiatric out-patient clinic, hospital casualty department or even GP surgery or domiciliary visit, the above information is often collected on the basis of one or two interviews. The value of community work engaging people with longer term experiences of distress is the ability to gradually build up a full picture of the client's background and circumstances, usually at a pace which is comfortable for the client. With good communication between different staff, the community setting can equal the in-patient setting for offering opportunities for collaboration, thus enabling a fuller assessment of mental state in the client's own environment.

Cautionary notes on the assessment of symptoms

The undertaking of a psychiatric interview has often been likened to a careful piece of detective work, but the inexperienced and overenthusiastic practitioner can easily fall into the trap of misinterpretation of the information observed. If the agenda is explicitly focused on the discovery of positive symptoms, one may overemphasize some observations and, equally important, unintentionally miss significant indications of other relevant information.

The client who has experienced severe mental distress over a long period of time is quite likely to have exhibited psychiatric symptoms on repeated occasions. With the exception of times when the client may be experiencing an acute episode of distress, the focus of mental health work is more productively engaged in an educative role – helping both client and significant carers to monitor and understand these experiences better themselves. This may frequently be a painstaking repetitive task, but the long-term rewards of providing more useful information to the client, and possibly encouraging a greater partnership for the future monitoring of symptoms, is well worth the effort of persistence.

Such a task can make productive use of basic counselling skills, working within the developing one-to-one relationship. The benefits of sharing experiences and knowledge through a group process should also be evaluated; clients, carers and mixed groups could be considered, but the individuals in this client group often experience greater difficulty managing the requirements of effective group work. Relapse, through the renewed or continuing experience of symptoms, may well be the norm before a client is able to demonstrate an appreciation of the educative information you are imparting, but this doesn't signify failure for either party.

The assessment of symptoms is not an end in itself. The medical model approach emphasizes the function of such an assessment in helping to formulate a diagnosis and indicate a course of treatment, but a good interview and assessment should also evaluate and respond to the client's own interpretation of the symptoms he or she is experiencing. In the case of distress to the client, or danger to the client or other people, rapid action is indicated. However, there are occasions when positive symptoms, such as grandiose delusions or second person auditory hallucinations, can be considered of desirable value or even companionship by the person experiencing them. We need to temper our haste to treat the person whose extreme social isolation is only broken by private conversations with their hallucinatory experiences. They may not thank you at a later date for depriving them of pleasant experiences and may become more difficult to engage in a further working relationship. It may be argued that the focus of attention on symptoms is what prevents the widening of the person's real social circumstances, but the alternative option should always be carefully considered rather than instantly dismissed as being against the norms of professional training.

The assessment of 'negative' symptoms presents a quite different problem for potential misinterpretation. The apparent presentation of neglect and apathy may, in fact, be a result of poor skills acquisition, or involve the more thorny area of intelligence where it can be extremely stigmatizing being labelled as 'low IQ'. Once again, the importance of building rapport to gain a clear history is indicated in order to make a more careful assessment of the current circumstances. It would also be of value to include the views of important carers and others in the history-taking and decision-making processes, wherever relevant.

PSYCHOSOCIAL INTERVENTIONS

Early warning signs of relapse

This area has been the focus of much attention in the recent development of community care. The community, as opposed to the hospital service, may offer better opportunities for monitoring and identifying the possible early warning signs and symptoms that may signify that a person is relapsing into a state of more severe distress. It is also of greater value to target the longer-term group of clients for such monitoring, on the basis that they have a longer history with more frequent occurrences of relapse and, it is generally considered, that the nature of the relapse will often take a slower and more insidious pattern than the incidents of acute episodes of distress. Changes in work and social function have been noted some months before the onset of acute symptoms of distress.

The focus of this work has taken a number of forms in research methodology, but we are, in practice, faced with the importance of good observation of mental state changes through visiting the client at home or through regular attendance at out-patient clinics. Again, the value of this type of work can only be considerably enhanced if we equip the client and significant carers with the relevant information to undertake their own monitoring of the changing situation in association with their professional workers. A note of warning at this point is that carers and clients will often take different views about the underlying causes of change. The worker involved in educating clients and carers needs to be aware of different focuses of attention and to make appropriate evaluations of information fed back from conflicting sources.

In the work to identify early warning signs of the relapse of an illness, two factors have been found to be frequently significant – the prominence of clearly identified life events during the period prior to relapse into severe distress (Birley and Brown, 1970) and the incidence of high expressed emotion in families (Leff and Vaughn, 1985). These are outlined by Bebbington and Kuipers (1988) as two of the main 'arousal theories of the onset and course of schizophrenia', which relate specifically to a person's sensitivity and responses to specific psychosocial stresses.

Life events

Many studies have been carried out to investigate this theory dating back to the late 1960s, but they were significantly expanded by Day *et al.* (1987) through a simultaneous study in nine centres world-wide, contrasting east and west, developed and underdeveloped cultures. The outcomes suggested significant results for six out of the nine centres relating to clusters of particular events arising in the period up to three weeks prior to the onset of illness.

However, the overall outcome of these studies still leaves many questions unanswered (Bebbington and Kuipers, 1988), particularly regarding the exact point of onset for a condition such as schizophrenia. At present there appears to be a more conclusive association between life events and depression than there is between life events and schizophrenia.

Examples of stressful life events considered in these studies include:

- significant losses through family bereavement or marital and relationship breakup;
- significant changes in housing, occupational status or financial status;
- potentially emotionally stressful events, e.g. birth of a child, marriage, Christmas.

Expressed emotion

The measure of expressed emotion includes a consideration of emotional over-involvement, criticism and hostility, and the associated poor levels of problem-solving skills. Tarrier *et al.* (1988a) suggest that it possibly operates via physiological arousal, pointing to the evidence from studies of skin conductance recordings, whereby high levels of conductance are specifically recorded when the subject is in the presence of a family member considered to exhibit high expressed emotion. Bebbington and Kuipers (1988) concluded that the overall evidence from wide-ranging studies strongly favours a causal role for expressed emotion in exacerbating the florid symptoms of schizophrenia.

The results of these many studies have focused on the development of behavioural family interventions to reduce the levels of expressed emotion through education, relative support groups or by reducing the amount of face-to-face contact in families (Tarrier *et al.* 1988b; Tarrier, 1990). Leff *et al.* (1987) concluded there is a strong association of good outcomes in schizophrenia with the development of beneficial family structures and traditions.

Some doubts have been cast on the outcomes of expressed emotion studies. Mechanic (1986) suggests they have had little impact on mental health practice. Birchwood *et al.* (1988) initiated a debate on the origins of expressed emotion, suggesting that it could grow as a natural reaction to a family having to cope with one of their own experiencing a condition such as schizophrenia.

Behavioural interventions

The social reactivity of schizophrenia is significant because it permits and encourages a constructive approach to the management of the condition (Bebbington and Kuipers, 1988). However, the development of family therapies needs to proceed with some caution because of the judgemental values it can occasionally give rise to. Particular attention should be drawn to suggestions that the individual may be symptomatic of wider family pathology or that specific family members, particularly women, should behave in identified caring roles (Williams and Watson, 1988).

Falloon, Boyd and McGill (1984) and Falloon *et al.* (1985) discuss the potential for the family management of schizophrenia through methods of behavioural social skills training to improve problem-solving skills in families. This involves learning to express positive feelings and a more constructive expression of negative feelings.

Tarrier (1991) has extended behavioural approaches to encompass the application of psychotherapeutic skills in the management of schizophrenia. It is argued that cognitive behavioural approaches can help to alleviate hallucinations, delusions and 'negative' symptoms of apathy and social withdrawal.

These interventions need to be evaluated and considered alongside the longer-standing physical treatments of the medical approach, particularly medication and ECT.

MEDICATION ISSUES

Since the first use of chlorpromazine for the treatment of psychiatric disturbance in 1951, medication has taken a central role in the medical management of severe mental distress. With regard to the treatment of schizophrenia using the major tranquillizer, Johnstone (1989) suggests that it offers no cure but may have some qualified success in suppressing distressing symptoms, helping people to live reasonable lives outside the hospital and preventing some relapse. But she also suggests these advantages are only accrued at some cost, which will be discussed further in this section.

Liberman *et al.* (1986) criticize the over-dependence of the psychiatric profession on medication, particularly as it has had little impact on the 'negative' symptoms such as apathy and withdrawal; the drugs have serious side-effects and do nothing to promote the survival skills necessary for living independently in the community. Mosher and Burti (1989) have pointed to a distinction between the proven effects of the major tranquillizer and the so-called mythical claims that remain unsubstantiated. For many people the long-term prognosis has remained unaltered with the advent of these drugs, though people with a particularly poor prognosis ultimately achieve degrees of acute symptom relief that may justify their use (Warner, 1985).

A general problem that arises in the wider consideration of treatment options is the battle between drug treatment and psychosocial alternatives. Mosher and Burti (1989) point out that the psychosocial interventions tend to be more complex, expensive and difficult to implement, though combinations of both may give rise to better outcomes (Johnson, 1988; Tarrier, 1990). The problem seems to be that medication-taking is a good reinforcer of the so-called 'sick role' and that one of the negative effects of drug-taking is its apparent block on the ability to engage in the demands of psychosocial intervention.

Administration of medication

The best choice of oral and/or intramuscular depot injection has been a matter for wide debate in the psychiatric profession. The advantages of the depot injection are generally presented in terms of the control it affords in monitoring compliance with medication regimes. It is also the only method of knowing exactly how much medication has been received when discussing the treatment of symptoms or side-effects. In the case of oral medication, the major advantage expressed is that of flexibility of prescription due to the shorter time period of its action.

From the point of view of clients in the long-term group, preference for administration of medication is equally varied, some preferring oral medication because of the flexibility of compliance/non-compliance that it affords them, others preferring injections rather than having to remember to take tablets a number of times each day. For many people the choice not to accept medication is generally frowned upon, particularly if it is exercised by those considered to be in the long-term group. It may even be seen as an example of illogical thought processes further indicating the underlying illness and need for medication.

Maintenance medication

The need for long-term maintenance medication remains unclear in the case of the first incidence of an illness, but the importance of maintenance neuroleptic treatment in the prevention of acute relapse and rehospitalization for longer-term histories of illness has been repeatedly demonstrated. However, Johnson (1988) does suggest that 'the decision to prescribe long-term maintenance neuroleptic therapy must be based on a careful evaluation of all known facts and the true risk–benefit ratio must be fully explored'. This needs an ongoing evaluation of the potential for developing disturbing extrapyramidal side-effects, occasionally progressing to the risks of developing tardive dyskinesia for people receiving neuroleptic medication continuously over a number of years.

Carpenter and Heinrichs (1983) have suggested that 'targeted drug treatment' can be used to treat symptoms as they arise, rather than using the idea of maintenance doses even when symptoms are not present. This could reduce the risks of developing progressively severe side-effects. However, this idea has only been considered successful in selected cases (Carpenter *et al.* 1990), and is not so applicable to many people in this long-term group (some of whom persistently exhibit symptoms). It is possible that the closer relationship of the case manager role could be quite beneficial for promoting the close monitoring of symptomatic change and variable use of medication (Onyett, 1992).

In its favour, maintenance medication for clients with long-term mental distress is considered to have a buffer effect

against stress and life events, either preventing a relapse or modi-
fying the consequences in a slightly more favourable way (Leff
and Vaughn, 1981). It is also widely felt that maintenance
medication provides some protection against the stresses involved
in participating in other forms of therapy – rehabilitation programmes, social therapy, psychotherapy, behaviour therapy or
occupational therapy. Johnstone (1989) points to a contradictory
view, that the taking of powerful sedatives inevitably results
in damaging apathy. This consequently undermines any
attempts to engage in programmes of social rehabilitation.

To its detriment, maintenance medication studies have been
unable to give specific indications as to the duration of time
a client should continue taking the drugs. It has been suggested
that a majority of patients will relapse when they stop taking
medication, even after compliance of five years or more
(Johnson, 1988). It would be reasonable to explore the possibility of negotiating regular, short, drug-free holidays to reduce
the total dosage and risk of side-effects in the many cases where
a person is recommended to take medication for such long
periods of time, often for life. Warner (1985) also draws attention to an extremely damaging condition of 'tardive psychosis'
which may result from withdrawal from a major tranquillizer,
causing a rebound to much more intense experiences of the
original symptoms. A further problem with maintenance
medication is its disturbing ability to alter a person's appearance, even before the degrees known as tardive dyskinesia.
The result can often be blank expressions, grimaces and a
shuffling gait.

Monitoring medication

The most reliable way a community service can monitor the
amount of medication taken is through the administration of
depot injections. But we cannot impose methods of treatment
on people purely for the purpose of efficient management from
the service providers point of view. In an ideal world, we
should provide sufficient information and support for a client
to understand the need for medication and to monitor their
own administration.

Mosher and Burti (1989) advocate that the ultimate decisions
about whether to take medication or not should rest with the

client. But this should be an informed choice based on the option for full information and support to monitor symptoms and side-effects on a close day-to-day basis. Services should be responsive to client and carer reports.

In reality, we also have a responsibility to safeguard against the hoarding of tablets for fear of overdose, intentional or otherwise. Particularly close supervision may be indicated where people have a previous history of depression, overdoses or difficulty following prescription instructions, especially when an individual may be prescribed a number of different types of medication together. This is an area that promotes the need for good collaboration, particularly between GP and psychiatrist. But there is often a valuable role to be played by the case manager in facilitating good channels of communication on a regular basis, through more frequent contact with the different medical practitioners.

For specific methods of monitoring the administration of medication, the dosett box and the pill mill have been devised. They are containers which have separate slots for each required dose according to times of the day and days of the week. Many clients are able to manage the use of these systems with a little advice and information. The refilling of these containers, usually on a weekly basis, may be carried out in a number of different ways. It may be adequate to supervise the client refilling the container from a pharmacy bottle supply held at home or, in some circumstances, the pharmacist may agree to refill the container directly, providing the repeat prescriptions are received from the GP. There is some controversy about the details of different workers' roles here: pharmacists can legally fill medication containers, some nursing staff are covered to do so, non-nursing staff are definitely not legally covered. Anybody may supervise the activity if it is physically performed by a client accepting such supervision.

In the case of old supplies of tablets, hoarded or suddenly discovered at home deliberately or accidentally, it is advisable to seek medical advice on their subsequent use or supervise their disposal – clients may flush small quantities down the lavatory or they may be returned to the pharmacy. When hoarding is suspected, it would be wise to be closely observant in the client's home, within the boundaries of home visiting etiquette, in case of the possible discovery of favoured hiding places. It would be inappropriate to search the home against the client's wishes, and the discovery of any hidden supplies should provide a basis for discussing the possible problems and organizing a domiciliary visit by a psychiatrist or a GP to help assess suicide potential if necessary.

In the case of Mary, in the previous case study, it also became necessary to lock supplies of tablets in a strong box, and for the visiting District Nurse to supervise the use of a dosett box on a daily basis rather than a weekly basis because of the risk of Mary taking an unintentional overdose.

Objections to medication

Some of these have already been raised in the discussion, directly or indirectly. However, the frequent experiences of people with long-term difficulties being required to accept long-term medication make the wide-ranging objections significant enough for separate consideration.

One of the most frequent reasons for objection, and subsequent promotion of non-compliance with the prescriptions, is the assumption that a person should surrender to long-term dependence on medication, even for life in many cases. Johnstone (1989) points to a failure by the medical profession to capitalize on the potential benefits to some people by simply failing to provide adequate explanations of why medication is needed, for how long, in what circumstances it can be reduced and what may be the potentially distressing side-effects. Failure to explain has even bordered on a disregard for the basic right to refuse for the majority of informally consenting patients.

Wing and Morris (1981) have suggested that people may not comply with prescribed medications on the grounds of not wishing to permit chemical agents into the body, that they may have an unwillingness to admit to long-term disability, or that they may even enjoy some of the positive symptoms, e.g. friendly hallucinations or feelings of power. However, they also suggest that the dislike of potential and actual side-effects remains a most significant objection to long-term use of medication.

Johnstone (1989) outlines an explanation of progressively distressing side-effects, from generalized feelings of restlessness, apathy, weight gain and blurred vision, to the more serious and potentially irreversible disabilities of pseudo-parkinsonism and tardive dyskinesia. In this latter condition, the person can adopt uncontrollable movements of the lip, tongue and face, fidgeting hands, tapping feet, rocking motions and other bizarre involuntary mannerisms. She also suggests that the risks of suffering these consequences are feared to be greater with the widespread practice of polypharmacy, whereby people are placed on combinations of major tranquil-lizer, receiving a variety of tablets in addition to a depot injection. There often appears to be a greater willingness in the psychiatric profession to prescribe more medication at higher doses than to consider the benefits of a drug-reducing regime in combination with other types of intervention. Johnstone (1989) fears the prominence of a 'try it and see' experimental approach to drug prescribing. Occasionally the needs of the service seem to outweigh the needs of the patient, with evidence that medications are prescribed in larger quantities on wards when there are pressures through staff shortages.

Ultimately, the stigma raised by the bizarre appearances induced by the prescription of medication (e.g. the Modecate shuffle) can be as debilitating as the stigma acknowledged against the appearances resulting from the experiences of illness itself. In many cases this cost proves to be high, particularly for those people where the experience of medica-tion, so far, has been one of only partial effectiveness in the control of symptoms.

Whatever the basis for the objections raised against the long-term use of medication, it is important that they are acknow-ledged constructively. Refusal should not be dealt with in a punitive manner or be seen as failure on the part of the professional worker. Though there is much evidence to suggest that medication can have positive effects for people experi-encing long-term distress (Johnson, 1988), its prescription should always be approached on an individual case-by-case consideration – always acknowledging the potential negative consequences (Johnstone, 1989) and the constant need for review and reduction, but above all else acknowledging the individual's right to exercise an informed choice (Mosher and Burti, 1989).

Greater compliance can only genuinely be advocated through a greater information-giving role. In this way, supportive counselling can then be used to weigh up the positive and negative consequences of taking prescribed medication, including the potential for relapse if medication is ceased. A stronger relationship can also provide the basis for negotiating medication reductions and drug-free periods, with the support of close monitoring by the client, carers and support workers (Onyett, 1992). (However, it is important to note that this is not presently the norm for people detained following serious offences, who continue under Home Office supervision, or other forms of compulsory detention under the Mental Health Act 1983. In these cases compliance with medication may frequently be made a condition of discharge from hospital.)

ECT (electroconvulsive therapy)

Johnstone (1989) provides a critical account of the uses of ECT as a treatment for cases of resistant mental illnesses, particularly severe depressive illness. She outlines the procedure, the debate over its potential effects on the brain, the official view that it is clearly demonstrated to be a rapidly effective treatment for severe depression, and reports the alternative critical account proposed by the American psychiatrist Peter Breggin.

Willis (1984) suggests that ECT is apparently the most successsful of physical treatments but that its mode of action remains unknown. He puts forward speculative suggestions that it may work through a process of alterations to central nervous system arousal and conditionability or perhaps by altering a central mood regulating system. Its detractors claim that ECT works more by 'shocking' patients into altering their own behaviour, and that perhaps the extra care and attention afforded as a precautionary measure with this treatment elicits its own improved responses.

Reports of concerns expressed by Breggin (Johnstone, 1989) present a disturbing account of its potential harm by creating a post-traumatic confusional syndrome, characterized by varying degrees and duration of memory loss and leading possibly to irreversible brain damage. In general texts, the concerns for memory loss and confusion tend to be minimized to minor consequences of short-term duration which the patient should be prepared for before administration of treatment.

Johnstone (1989) finds it difficult to be objective in the face of such conflicting views. She suggests that maybe it succeeds by removing negative memories (as well as the positive) and through relieving guilt feelings by its associations of punishment. Willis (1984) suggests there may be as high as an 85% success rate in the rapid reduction of depressive symptoms when treated with ECT. He moves closer to the views expressed by its detractors when discussing the high relapse rates, which often requires subjects to be considered for repeated courses of treatment.

With such inconclusive and conflicting evidence, Johnstone (1989) concludes that ECT can only be considered as truly effective for people experiencing high-risk, life-threatening cases of severe depression. Its use with schizophrenia is far more controversial (Willis, 1984). Dr Anthony Clare has been reported to suggest that ECT is a much more abused and over-used method of treatment because it is so much easier and quicker to implement than the complex psychosocial interventions (Johnstone, 1989). Its use as an out-patient treatment can only be assumed to add to the potential over-use.

SUPPORTING THE USE OF MEDICAL SERVICES

Liaison

As the central figure in providing support, with the likelihood of the most frequent contact, a case manager is in a position to build the strongest relationship with, and acquire the most knowledge of, the client.

In building a network of support to meet the client's needs, he or she may also provide the strongest links in the structure – facilitating communication between the client and medical services, and between the different services themselves.

This liaison role often involves substantial amounts of groundwork to promote the delivery of services necessary to meet the client's specific needs, such as regular communication with the GP, psychiatrist, community psychiatric nurse and others. Good communication between all services is essential for promoting a positive environment of collaboration towards the common goal of offering the most appropriate services for meeting the client needs.

Out-patient appointments

Many people experiencing long-term mental distress will have been offered periodic out-patient appointments at a psychiatric clinic. If these appointments are with a consultant psychiatrist, the client may be seeing the same individual regularly, with whom he or she may establish a relationship. If they are seen by a junior doctor working with the consultant, the likelihood is that they will be seen by a series of different people. The number of visits to the same doctor will be determined by the frequency of appointments and how often the doctor's placements rotate. As a consistent support worker your attendance at the appointment may be widely appreciated – the client may value the moral and practical support from a familiar person and the psychiatrist should value the knowledge of a professional who knows the person well.

Inconsistency of personnel may be the one reason why clients drop out of contact with the out-patient clinic. Whatever the reason for non-attendance, the community support worker may be able to offer valuable advice and education to encourage a client to re-establish contact if the professionals involved consider further attendance to be of some value to the clients.

Domiciliary visits

There are many and varied reasons for medical practitioners (GP and/or psychiatrist) to visit a client at home. The client may wish support but feels unable to attend the clinic, it may be at the carers' request, or it may be that the case manager has some specific concerns about the client's health requiring a medical opinion. Whatever the particular reason, the case manager will be required to do the liaising to arrange a visit and to accompany the medical practitioner during the visit. This is likely to require preparation of the client and carers about the nature, purpose and likely outcome of the arranged visit, e.g. reassurance that compulsory admission may or may not be likely.

Extended hours and emergency services

One of the significant criticisms levelled against the developing community care services is their availability only during short periods of time, often only the 37 hours normal office time. Occasionally flexible working hours may increase availability, but at a reduced level of service. Even at best, two-thirds of a client's week would not be covered, with evenings and week-ends frequently quoted as times of particular vulnerability.

There is a strong case for each individual service to evaluate the possibility of extended hours in relation to local need. The arguments to be considered are that supply may reveal previously unmet needs as well as appropriate and possibly inappropriate demands on a particular service. This could subsequently focus a stronger reliance on 'mental health' services rather than encouraging the wider use of community resources. Furthermore, it is arguable whether the resources of small teams spread even more thinly would improve the level of service offered, particularly to the long-term client group who are deemed in need of more intensive levels of support. While the needs of the services should not be placed above the needs of the clients, these points should be very carefully examined in relation to the assessed needs and wishes of the client group. The issue of adequate staff support and potential burn-out is a further factor to be considered before deciding to extend a service.

In the absence of extended hours coverage, the case manager should be responsible for informing and educating the clients and carers about the availability of the normal emergency services and any other emergency mental health services in the area such as:

- on-call GP services;
- duty psychiatrist through a hospital emergency clinic or casualty department;
- emergency duty social worker systems;
- voluntary services, e.g. Samaritans;
- initiatives in self-advocacy (see Chapter 9).

LEGISLATIVE ISSUES

As indicated in the introductory chapter, the legal and legislative issues in mental health are a large area not able to be covered adequately in this text. However, I wish to draw your attention to two significant issues which will impinge on the role of the case manager, both of which will reflect the continuing need for close links between the community services and the hospital services.

From community into hospital

The area of involuntary admission to psychiatric hospitals arouses great debate in the field of mental health, including significant opposition from the 'user movement' (see Chapter 9).

It would not be appropriate to cover the mechanics of the 1983 Mental Health Act at this point, but to let us examine the role the case manager can play in attempting to minimize the distress when the circumstances are such that one of your clients is being admitted to hospital under compulsory detention. Primarily, this will take the form of an advocacy role because the case manager has no statutory role in this respect, as compared with the GP, psychiatrist or approved social worker.

In addition to the distress experienced by clients or carers as a result of the mental health difficulties, further distress may be unintentionally caused by the organization of the process. Though it is difficult to co-ordinate the timetables of a number of different people, the client is quite suddenly faced with several people unfamiliar to him or her and, occasionally, a potentially upsetting police presence. The circumstances of the need for a mental health section may dictate the need for particular tactics, but the case manager can advocate for the most careful consideration of the situation – this should, hopefully, be the client agreeing to accompany one or two people into hospital by normal transport (car or taxi) or accepting another solution such as taking medication at home with regular monitoring by professional staff. Failing this, an ambulance with minimal police presence is preferable, to enable a safe admission with a minimum of distress.

The case manager then assumes the important responsibility of maintaining visits to ensure continuity through community and hospital care. This should include ensuring ongoing discussions of patients' rights to enable a fuller understanding of the situation, by engaging the support of self-advocacy groups where available and initiating progressive discharge plans through attendance at ward rounds and meetings. The case manager can provide the vital link to ensure that needs outside the hospital are appropriately addressed while the person is an in-patient, e.g. bills and debts, benefit entitlements, furnishing and cleaning in the home.

From hospital back to community

Section 117 of the 1983 Mental Health Act states the need for health authorities and local authorities to make suitable provision of after-care services for patients that have been detained under section 3 or 37 of the same Act. In relevant cases, this legislation may require the case manager to be specifically involved in the negotiations of such services before the point of discharge.

The legislative procedures of Section 117 are limited by statute to a range of patients who have been detained under specific sections of the 1983 Mental Health Act. However, the 'Care Programme' approach should now extend similar provisions to all people discharged from psychiatric units after April 1991. This approach has been embodied in the government White Paper *Caring for People* (1989), but its origins are traced back through a number of reports to the Social Services Committee Report of 1985 (Ryan, Ford and Clifford, 1991). In essence, the health and social needs of all psychiatric patients should be assessed before discharge, with a plan of implementation, a process of review and a named responsible worker (who may come from any agency). The White Paper indicates that a 'case manager' be nominated in cases where needs are complex and significant levels of resources involved.

Although the responsible workers can be nominated from any agency, it would be reasonable to assume that the community services will be expected to carry a significant amount of responsibility for monitoring and reviewing such plans. The White Paper does indicate a need to improve patients' quality of life through plans that are realistic in terms of staffing and the community services available – herein lies an acknowledgement that there may be a gap between expectations and available resources. Substantial new resources would be needed, particularly if the plans to extend the legislation to all discharged patients are to be put into practice.

SUMMARY

The focus of concern in this chapter is to promote an understanding of how the medical impairments of long-term mental health problems manifest themselves in the community. Particular attention is drawn to the changing needs and patterns of providing support in the community as opposed to institutional settings.

Two particular debates are addressed; firstly, the debate on the hospital versus the community as the better care and support environment for people experiencing long-term severe distress. This should not be allowed to gravitate towards a polarized debate. Pilling (1991) illustrates the process of change but maintains the importance of the hospital as an individual aspect of the community service rather than an isolated alternative. The psychiatrist, whether still based in the hospital or in community multi-disciplinary teams, should provide the specialist support to an increasingly important primary care service focused around the GP (Shepherd *et al.* 1981).

The second debate centres around the questions of medical care and psychosocial care. The views of Dr Anthony Clare (in Johnstone, 1989) expressed on ECT may well echo the wide provision of physical treatments, suggesting they are over-used simply because they are quicker and easier to resort to than the more complex psychosocial interventions, particularly if services are pressured into the need for rapid results and quick turnovers.

Despite widespread criticisms of a purely medical approach (Johnstone, 1989), even the detractors have sometimes concluded that physical treatments have more relevance to the more chronic group (Warner, 1985). Most psychiatrists are now of the opinion that an eclectic approach should involve physical treatments supporting the progress with other forms of intervention (Johnson, 1988).

Mosher and Burti (1989) are much more in favour of individual client choice, including the use of medication. They favour the benefit of much greater information-giving and offers of close monitoring and support to facilitate genuine informed choices. Much broader scope for interventions with individuals and their families (Tarrier, 1990; 1991) should open up wider choices. Onyett (1992) advocates a strong role for case managers to help in the promotion of greater individual choice. Through the close relationship and frequency of contact there is a genuine opportunity for providing more information and supporting better monitoring of changes in the client.

5

Housing

The most crucial aspect of any strategy to follow the approach of developing care in the community must be the provision of adequate accommodation. Suitable housing tends to be the highest priority need expressed by clients themselves. It is a basic human need for all of us and provides the essential base from which we take on the further challenges of maintaining meaningful occupation and social connections.

For people experiencing long-term severe distress, the first half of the twentieth century offered only permanent incarceration in mental institutions. As this option was increasingly seen as being inappropriate, a rapid growth of different community-based residential services took place. More and more people were being located in mini-institutions, board and lodgings, hostels, bed and breakfast, living with family, or found among the destitute and poor in shelters, prisons or on the street. As recently as 1985, the House of Commons Social Services Committee has been reporting that the provision and co-ordination of community residential options is clearly inadequate when compared with the pace of closure of the large mental hospitals.

Much of what is provided up to now tends to result from a deficits or problems approach to assessing need. There is a negative assumption that many people have a limited capacity to function and will require a very high level of staff support; consequently, the bricks and mortar are arranged to suit service needs rather than client needs. McAusland (1985) has suggested that we have a great deal of experience in accommodating very large numbers of people, 100–1000+, in psychiatric hospitals; we have a fair amount of experience of hostels and nursing homes accommodating 10–40 people; we also have a fair amount of experience accommodating smaller numbers in group homes; but what we most lack, in the British psychiatric experience, is the support for people with major and long-term disabilities in ordinary housing.

Wing and Morris (1981) have succinctly outlined the needs of the mentally ill from non-hospital residential accommodation, and in most respects they are the problems shared by the general population – reasonable accommodation at a price that can be afforded with some protection from housing-related stress through excessive charges by unscrupulous landlords, insecurity of tenure, poor maintenance and repair. Other needs expressed included a sensitive balance of independence and support, tolerance of unusual behaviour patterns and erratic payments, and help with some of the practical tasks of daily living.

Whereas some of the needs expressed may be specific to a client group, Howat *et al.* (1988) indicate that

housing for the chronically mentally ill cannot be considered in isolation from general housing policy and the operations of the benefit system any more than it can from the ability of health, social services and voluntary organisations to provide appropriate care and support. Unfortunately the current policies, preoccupations, and endeavour of these agencies are disjointed, and this has prevented the emergence of an integrated view of how services should develop.

Many individual writers have recently concluded that better co-ordinated policies are required so that each person may have the choice of suitable housing with support arranged to meet individual need (Heginbotham, 1985a; Garety, 1988; Pilling, 1991). Whether being discharged from an institution or already resident in the community, support services should be flexible enough to meet changing needs and situations; clients can then remain in their favoured home and not necessarily be expected to move to a different home that could better suit their changed circumstances. Whilst the option of more supported accommodation, in the form of homes and hostels, should still ideally be available, the over-riding principle governing housing policy should be the right of self-determination, where the notion of 'choice' replaces that of 'placement' (Garety, 1988). We must be particularly aware of the psychologically positive aspects of having a place that can be referred to as 'home' and not just a place that provides the most basic function of shelter.

Throughout this chapter, I propose to look at the relationship between housing and mental health and briefly survey the options that have been provided for people with persistent severe distress, including more especially the range of support services that may be flexibly provided for people in their own separate homes. However, any discussion of housing provision for people with mental health problems cannot ignore the question of homelessness and mental health.

HOMELESSNESS AND MENTAL HEALTH

The continued evidence of homeless people on the streets of all major cities remains a politically charged issue, rife with argument and counter argument and always backed up with a range of mesmerizing statistics. I have no intention of trying to propose any solutions in this text, but it remains relevant to reiterate the incidence of chronic mental health problems consistently identified in any surveys of the homeless. Such high incidences need to be kept in mind when considering the allocation, management and support policies being pursued in the housing of people with the experience of severe mental distress. In fact, Pilling (1991) suggests that some of these practices may even have contributed to the numbers of homeless mentally people, through ill-considered and poorly co-ordinated discharge policies.

The figures are quite alarming. Garety (1988) suggests that between 25% and 50% of homeless people living in hostels and shelters have recently been discharged from psychiatric hospitals in the UK. This figure presumably does not include the many others experiencing severe distress, including the street homeless who have had no specific contact with specialist psychiatric services. In the USA, Bachrach and Nadelson (1988) report varying estimates, from 30% to 90%, of the homeless population of different cities suffering from chronic mental conditions – including long duration, frequent recurrence and a progressive degree of seriousness of their condition. This they suggest is often combined with a chronic physical condition.

Part of the problem stems from the widely held attitude that homeless people who have special needs must be a danger to themselves, a danger to others and constitute an unsightly problem which would be better kept out of sight. Part of the problem also stems from the inadequate statutory responses to these misguided perceptions, resulting in people being directed into large institutional hostels, prison or run-down accommodation, with little in the way of appropriate support being included in the package. The housing legislation outlines a duty for local authority housing departments to rehouse single homeless people who are considered to be vulnerable within the terms of the Acts (1985 Housing Act), with the intention of establishing some housing rights for those people least able to compete for secure housing outside of the public sector (Brough and Craig, 1985). However, it has been found that many of the so-called vulnerable people do not even arrive at the starting point – the Homeless Persons Unit – because they perceive the system to be oblivious to their particular needs and unlikely to do anything for them other than directing them to the aforementioned institutional options.

Hirst (1988) suggests that

> because the system does not address either long-term housing or support needs, people tend to drift in and out of services which reinforce their homelessness, without access to the same medical and support services the home based community has. Lack of specialist support is not the only reason for this worsening situation; the overall housing crisis, and the shortage of appropriate permanent housing for people with special needs have also had an impact.

Despite the evidence of homeless people with special needs losing out on the services they need, there is very little agreement about how these needs should be met in the future. The predominant solution is still one of providing separate services, usually in the form of hostels or bed and breakfast accommodation allocated specifically for vulnerable homeless people. Little consideration seems to be given to the stresses such a placement may have on an already vulnerable person, and scant consideration for the support which may be required.

Only recently are we beginning to see patchy attempts to prioritize the need for appropriate support, even if the location of the accommodation remains the same (Brent-Smith and Dean, 1990). The focus of this text, on a case-management style of outreach and co-ordination, is now seen as being equally appropriate for assessing and starting to meet the complex needs of the homeless people experiencing long-term mental health problems. The value of the multi-disciplinary team approach is being seen in the assessment and provision of support to people in some of London's large hostels (Timms and Fry, 1989); and a similar approach has been adopted by the New York 'street outreach teams' (Bachrach and Nadelson, 1988). Once again, the message is one of providing a person-alized support service for individuals, for people with complex multiple difficulties, and not with the aim of devising a uniform answer to meet the needs of an homogeneous population.

THE RELATIONSHIP OF HOUSING TO MENTAL HEALTH

Housing should be seen as one of the most necessary components when considering the care and support being offered to a person suffering long-term mental health problems (Heginbotham, 1985a). All too often a rehabilitation plan is drawn up for an individual, with only a passing assumption that the eventual placement will be suitable for the plan to be implemented. The ultimate location may only be determined by what is available at the time, with the pressure on hospital beds taking a higher priority than individual housing need. Kay and Legg (1986) found that many discharged hospital patients did not return to their previous address, had little involvement in any choices or decisions and that most were generally unsatisfied with the accommodation they found themselves placed in.

Even in the apparently progressive services, where housing need is professionally assessed and served by a wide range of provision, the person suffering with long-term difficulties is likely to face an obstacle course on a par with the Grand National horse race. The individual may express a desire for a flat in ordinary housing, but he or she could be confronted with the need to successfully transfer from hospital ward to hospital-hostel, to supported group home, to shared flat, to their own flat. A study of the concept of 'life events' will show that moving house is a very stressful event. We all feel stressed when we have to relocate in our own lives, yet a person who is vulnerable to emotional pressures is required to make a whole series of transitions before they may achieve their personal aim. Pressure indeed! Are we not setting up an already emotionally stressed individual to almost certain failure?

The notion that there may be connections between mental health problems and the range of housing issues to do with policy, housing conditions and specific housing problems, has not received the study that it deserves. Etherington (1983) outlines the research into the main theories of stress or drift – does bad housing contribute stresses to the onset of mental illness or do people with mental health problems drift into circumstances of multiple deprivation? Inconclusively, there are some suggestions that the stress theory holds up more in the case of depressive illnesses and the drift theory is more applicable to the occurrence of psychotic illnesses such as schizophrenia. But real life circumstances are far too complex to fit into such neatly defined categories.

Specific housing problems and conditions are felt to have some influence on precipitating illness and relapse, but again the research evidence tends to be inconclusive (Etherington, 1983):

- living on housing estates, particularly in high-rise flats – it has been suggested that social isolation and the lack of garden space can contribute to stress;
- overcrowding is considered to cause stress through the associated decreased privacy;
- noise and inter-tenant disputes contribute to stress and some feelings of persecution;
- cold and damp housing conditions and/or infestations contribute to stress through reduced habitable space and subsequent overcrowding and reduced privacy.

Whilst it may be argued that it is difficult initially to prevent the bad housing conditions or stigmatized attitudes of neighbours to a person suffering from the many manifestations of long-term distress, housing services could adopt a policy which attempts to avoid relocating a recovering individual in conditions that may have contributed to the original distress. A policy of offering 'hard-to-let' tenancies to people vulnerable to stress will hardly promote good practices or preventative measures.

Though ideally we should all actively promote the notion of client choice, the finer details of demand for housing at the individual level is very complex. Whether a person's perception of his or her housing-related stress is accurate and fears of persecution real or delusional, and whether a professional assessment accurately reflects real demand, the final outcome is always going to be one of different choices for different people and changing patterns of demand over time. The evidence to date suggests that the wants expressed by people and the needs expressed by professionals vary greatly (Kay and Legg, 1986).

In reality, the economics of supply will tend to overrule the principle of a demand-led service. A constant criticism of the overall shift from institutions to community is that the former outstrips the latter in its pace of progress, particularly if we look at the need for suitable accommodation for people discharged from the institutional care of the large hospitals. It is often the case that if a place is available in supported accommodation, the staff assessments of need will lead to placement with little regard for the personal choice of the client. 'Hard-to-let' tenancies are often offered in order to offset the alternative to homelessness or to avoid a long and stressful wait for a more suitable tenancy. All too often mental health and housing factors are not linked sufficiently and placement tends to rule over personal 'choice'.

Perhaps the most significant failure, in these circumstances, is that of overlooking the distinction between a housing 'need' and a housing 'want' or desire. The psychologically positive aspects of helping a person to achieve the security and stability of a home will then be lost.

An understanding of the economics of the housing market should not lead us to simply accept unsatisfactory situations. We have a responsibility to redress the inadequacies of the whole complex system. The following personal profile and case studies are included at this point to illustrate some of the inconsistencies that arise in the complex interactions between the responsibilities of health, social services and housing authorities. These are not isolated or extreme examples.

PERSONAL PROFILE

Pete is a 34-year-old man, born in England, with his parents originating in Dominica. His parents divorced while Pete was still very young and he lived with the family of his mother's second marriage. In addition to his stepfather he also has a younger stepbrother and stepsister, but these relationships have tended not to be developed.

Pete is described as being an intelligent and hard-working child. He left school with 'O' level passes and subsequently achieved Stage I Bookkeeping and Accounts qualifications at a local college. He built up a reasonable work record between the ages of 16 and 25, including three years in bench joinery and a further three years using his bookkeeping skills as a British Rail booking clerk. He also engaged in a close relationship, from his late teenage years, by which a daughter was born when Pete was 21.

It was during his mid-20s that Pete began to experience a progressive social and emotional decline. The most significant aspects of this process are the loss of his partner and child, no further employment since the age of 25 and increasingly aggressive conflicts with a family that have continued to offer practical support. A dramatic drift into personal and social neglect, distancing him from former friendships, has also been accompanied by use of illegal drugs, frequent contact with the legal system and subsequent referrals to the psychiatric services.

Pete attributes his recent difficulties to the physical affects of a motor-cycle accident. He was only considered to need a brief assessment and discharge without hospital admission at the time. His neglectful, defensive and sometimes aggressive behaviour patterns are generally attributed to an underlying schizophrenic illness. Following three brief admissions to psychiatric hospital, there are few recorded factors that support a definite diagnosis of his condition. He is considered to generally suffer from the negative manifestations of such an illness with little evidence of active symptoms. Although Pete is believed to respond quite positively to anti-psychotic medication when admitted to hospital, he has never had any desire to comply with medical treatments immediately from the point of discharge.

Avoidance of contact seems to be Pete's main pre-occupation when discharged from hospital. This has often included contact with his other family members – he will approach their home if he is in need of money, but generally repels their approaches to his home by confusing or sometimes aggressive gestures. He is known to have had neighbourly disputes, some of which appear to be the result of his reactions to people and some of which appear to be his reaction to the initial actions of others interfering with his privacy. He has also been asked to leave his one brief encounter with a day unit, allegedly on the grounds of threatening behaviour to other users and attempted theft. Pete generally exercises control over the contact statutory agency workers can have in their efforts to support him by more frequently not answering the door to visitors.

In terms of housing, since the beginning of his period of social decline Pete has managed a number of local council tenancies, and brief experiences of direct-access hostels. He has been repeatedly resettled through the efforts of the council special needs resettlement team. His ability to cope with such tenancies is frequently called into doubt because of the nature of his neighbourly disputes, his loss of keys, leaving his front door open and vulnerable to thefts, non-payment of bills, an accidental fire and general neglect of himself and the property. He frequently acknowledges a need for support but more often avoids or fails to complete the actions he is advised to take. He has generally resisted the offers of considering more supported accommodation, preferring to find other reasons why particular problems arise, with a suggestion that they will not reoccur in a subsequent tenancy. But they invariably do, in one form or another.

Pete is an example of somebody who requests ordinary housing and is repeatedly given ordinary housing with offers of support but who repeatedly indicates a failure to cope with such housing or use the support offered. In a professional sense, he appears to be an individual who could benefit from a brief period of skills development in a slightly more supported form of accommodation. To the credit of the services, his needs are reflected back to him but his wants still continue to take precedence.

Positive characteristics

- He is clear and consistent about his own requirements.
- He is capable of controlling the level of support he receives from other people.
- He is consistent about his longer-term aim to use his past strengths to gain future occupational status, but realistic about his current abilities.
- He uses a well-developed survival instinct in apparently poor life circumstances.

Pete's own expression of needs:

- to return to studying for further bookkeeping qualifications to support his future return to employment;
- a better source of income than his current invalidity benefit from social security benefits;
- a new tenancy in a better part of the borough;
- to re-establish contact with his long lost daughter.

CASE STUDY

Accommodating an institutionalized lifestyle

George is a 67-year-old man, previously discussed in Chapter 4. Since the age of 33 his experiences of mental health problems have resulted in his being placed in a long succession of institutionalized forms of supported living, beginning with four admissions to a long-stay psychiatric hospital ranging from four years to nine years in duration. Successive professional assessments of housing needs have indicated the suitability of high-care supported hostels, with George being referred to aftercare mental health hostels each time he has been discharged from hospital; except on the first, and shortest, period of community resettlement when he was offered board and lodgings.

On each occasion George has settled into a very minimal lifestyle centred around a kettle, an ashtray and a radio, with the active symptoms of his illness to plague him on a constant basis. The final hospital discharge in 1982 resulted in a settled period of a six-year residence in a particular staffed hostel, which eventually evicted him for disturbing other residents by playing his radio through the night. This resulted in five days of street homelessness until he was directed to a Salvation Army men's hostel. He remained there for 18 months, until he could be resettled by his case manager in a suitable, smaller, staffed mental after-care hostel.

The dilemma for George is his reliance on professional assessments of his housing needs and suitable placement. In extensive discussions to elicit his wants, he is more concerned with accommodating his particular interests than he is in the 'bricks and mortar' – to smoke, drink tea, listen to the radio and have a local pub that will not be concerned about his poor self-care skills are all he seeks as distractions from the 'voices'. In this respect the assessment is simple, but finding a placement that will be 'permissive' rather than being unduly concerned with rehabilitation and behaviour modification is more of a problem.

CASE STUDY 2

The learning process towards independence

Yasim is a 26-year-old man of Moroccan origin who has lived in Britain since the age of six when his parents decided to set up home here. He has been medically diagnosed as suffering a schizophrenic illness since the age of 18 and has always lived at home with his parents. He has an older brother and two younger sisters, each of whom have experience of living independently in a flat.

The time had come for Yasim to seek his own independence, partly because of parental pressure for him to leave

at this most recent development, we should briefly consider the residential services developed over the last few decades which still provide the mainstay of public service provision to people in this client group.

Hostel-ward (hospital-hostel)

Hostel-wards were a development of the 1970s to accommodate the people perceived as being the most needy – the 'new long-stay'. These units were designed to accommodate between 10 and 20 residents, providing 24-hour nursing care. They were closely linked with the hospital services and occasionally organized to share the nursing staff of the local hospital. The two most widely known examples are the Maudsley on-site facility (Wykes, 1982) and Douglas House, an example of an off-site facility (Goldberg *et al.*, 1985).

A principal criticism against the hostel-ward is the ease with which institutional practices can render them little more than an improvement on the psychiatric hospital ward (Segal and Moyles, 1979). However, Garety and Morris (1984) suggest evidence that these units can promote positive client-orientated practices through good staff support and development. As they are a long-term home for many of the residents, their design and organization should reflect this status above the clinical functions. Close association with a local hospital enables easy transfer for a patient in great need, but equally important is the small number of residents who become capable of moving on to less supported accommodation.

Mental after-care hostels

Hostels accommodating in excess of 20 residents have been a common feature of community residential provision since the policy for closing the large psychiatric hospitals came into being. More recently they have been undergoing a change of emphasis, from high levels of nursing care to staffing by residential social workers. This change of staffing has also been accompanied by changing policy on length of stay, progressively towards a more rehabilitative function with a shorter stay. The philosophy of supporting people to achieve higher levels of independence, moving to their own accommodation with a possible return to employment, is believed to make these hostels often less suitable for the more disabled client group. Pilling (1991) outlines surveys which point to the difficulties that these hostels face in terms of offering successful rehabilitation practices. But there have also been some successes. Staff frustration is often expressed about individuals who block spaces by their inability to move on. However, many still retain a more permissive environment and can aid integration into local communities by minimizing institutional practices. Appropriate staffing and support can also enable some such hostels to manage more acute periods of distress without the need for a person to be admitted to hospital.

Group homes

Group homes were a popular residential development of the 1950s and 1960s in an attempt to tackle the stigma associated with institutional care. They have varied in size from three to eight places, where people have their own single bedroom with shared communal rooms and an expectation of supporting the sharing of daily living skills. Because of the closer approximation to family homes, the group home has been seen as more suited to the needs of an older clientele, with stable medical conditions, who wish to achieve a settled future; they are generally seen as less suited to the needs of a younger, more disturbed, clientele with less organized views of their future (Wing and Morris, 1981).

The group homes were set up with varying degrees of staff supervision. More recently they have been seen as possibly offering a smaller version of the hospital-hostel, by using higher levels of care to accommodate the needs of a more disabled group of clients. One of the criticisms has been that low staffing levels and supervision has often resulted in underactive and institutionalized residents (Ryan, 1979).

Sheltered accommodation

Sheltered units offer independent flats within a larger block, with shared day-room facilities. They are characterized by a front line of supervision through wardens and alarm systems in each flat to call for assistance if needed. Such services generally associated with a more elderly and physically frail client group and to date, little use is made of such facilities for people with severe mental health difficulties. Their suitability could be improved by the provision of outside specialist support services.

Nursing homes

These were generally established to cater for a more elderly and more chronic client group experiencing multiple physical frailities and in need of 24-hour nursing attention, although, on rare occasions, somebody younger than the usually considered elderly category of over 60 for women and 65 for men may be accommodated. Placement is usually for life, with the concern being one of care and attention rather than rehabilitation towards greater independence. Many nursing homes are run by the private sector, complementing the public sector Part III accommodation administered by local authority social services departments.

Boarding-out schemes/hostels/guest houses/ landlady schemes

These tend to be commercially operated schemes that can offer experience of catering for residential guests, and often require close supervision because of their variable responses to the care of people experiencing severe mental distress (Olsen, 1979).

DELIVERING INDIVIDUAL PACKAGES OF SUPPORT

We should not lose sight of the notion that community care aims to redress the institutional characteristic of separateness. We should not be seeking to highlight people's differences by congregating them into psychiatric ghettoes (Murray, 1978). An emphasis on a high need for professional supervision also tends to ignore the many people who have always found themselves coping with severe mental distress in ordinary housing, usually living with relatives. A flexible system of provision should see services revolving around the needs of the client in an ordinary home rather than an expectation that

the client will move from one location to another as a response
to their own changing levels of need (Gabell and Bevan, 1985).
Such an idea of 'floating support' places the emphasis of
flexibility and structural change firmly with the services rather
than expecting flexibility to be a function only for the client.
It envisages the possibility of a client becoming relatively
independent in the same place where they may have previously been highly supported.

McAusland (1985) clearly summarizes the challenge faced
by progressive community care services thus:

> It is important to stress that a residential service using
> ordinary housing does not mean dumping people without
> adequate support or discharging them without continuing
> access to skilled staff and services. Living in an ordinary
> house is not a cure for schizophrenia or any other psychiatric
> illness. From the knowledge that we have of the major
> mental illnesses we know that in many cases there will be
> a need for long-term, perhaps life-long support, assistance
> and treatment, and for help in recurrent crises. The
> challenge is whether we can deliver the intensity, variety
> and consistency of professional input to help someone to
> live in the mainstream of society in an ordinary house or
> flat despite their psychiatric disabilities and their continuing
> need for support'.

In reality, the challenge is one of moving away from the
medical notion of support which emphasizes the monitoring
of the progress of a person's illness to the co-ordination of a
diffuse and unstructured network of support, possibly involving many individuals and agencies from the formal health,
social and housing services, as well as the informal support
of friends, relatives and the local community (Nisbet, 1985;
Lovett, 1985).

The 'core and cluster' model

'Core and cluster' is a system for providing residential services
for people with long-term mental health problems, with a
flexible arrangement for adjusting support as individuals needs
change. The 'cluster' may be a range of different houses, flats
and bedsits offering a wide range of choice of housing options

in a local area. The 'core' is the administrative centre which forms the staff base from which they travel to offer support in the cluster houses. It is widely accepted that the core should not include any accommodation, such as a staffed hostel, in order to uphold the principle of separating accommodation and support functions. It is intended that this model can provide suitable accommodation for as long as desired, without subjecting the individual to multiple disruptive moves from one location to another (McAusland, 1985; Bayliss, 1987).

The House of Commons Social Services Committee (1985) suggested that although many references had been made to the idea of 'core and cluster' they still amounted to no more than words on paper, with very little in the way of schemes in operation. Indeed, project funding and housing management responsibilities have generally been left open to interpretation on a local basis, with the result that small schemes have tended to evolve in isolation as a result of local initiatives (Nisbet, 1985; Howat *et al.*, 1988).

Ordinary housing

Rather than looking to the complexity of combining housing management and support services under one body, such as the health authority, social services or a consortium of representatives from local services across all sectors, a wider approach has simply involved separating the housing and support functions to be provided by those who specialize in each.

In most local areas of the UK, the local authority housing department and a range of housing associations are likely to own and manage the stock of public sector housing. As specialists in the functions of allocating and managing housing units, it seems reasonable to rest such responsibilities where they most easily belong. Similarly, the health authority and local authority social services department will hold the expertise in offering support to those experiencing severe mental distress.

Within the guidelines of legislation and policy, the problem can be more clearly devolved down to local team level. Thus the housing officers and special needs resettlement officers on the one hand, and the providers of community support on

the other can be encouraged to collaborate more closely in order
to effectively meet the needs of individual clients. Each will
be more aware of the different roles, skills and responsibilities,
and each will have equal potential to act as advocates on the
client's behalf to the other services.

Under successive Housing Acts, local authority housing
departments have a duty to rehouse people considered to be
homeless, vulnerable and having a local connection, including
people experiencing severe mental distress, when they are
being discharged from hospital to community. Such duties are
generally initiated through the Homeless Persons Unit and
special needs housing resettlement teams of the local authority
(Brough and Craig, 1985). It is strongly recommended that
members of these teams and community support teams
develop strong links to better co-ordinate the service of
housing provision to the client. However, it is important to
note that not all local authorities have set up special needs
resettlement teams. Where they do exist, they are provided
as an additional service to meet local need, not as a statutory
requirement.

In conjunction with housing officers, the resettlement
worker may play an important part in the function of housing allocation, through a careful assessment of needs and a
consideration of suitable housing stock and location. This may
also include considering the geographical patches of the teams
that may be providing the ongoing support to an individual.
The resettlement worker may play a vital part in the most
unsettling first few months that a person takes up residence
– helping to adjust to the changes, taking on new skills,
attending to the necessary matters of claiming benefits, registering with a local G.P., discussing tenancy agreements, paying
rent and understanding the circumstances in which a tenancy
may be withdrawn, helping arrange connection of gas and
electricity services, and organizing any necessary repairs to
the property. Some of these functions may ultimately be
negotiated between client, resettlement worker and case
manager. The latter will certainly be expected to take on more
as the resettlement worker gradually withdraws after about
six months, though part of the negotiation may occasionally
involve the resettlement worker maintaining limited contact
or open access to advice from their specialist knowledge.

The function of longer-term housing management will shift more to the housing officer responsible for the property, estate or neighbourhood and, in some cases, to housing association staff if the local authority adopts a system of making nominations to them. Again, the case manager will need to maintain close contact in order to advocate on the client's behalf or negotiate involvement in effective housing management. Similarly, it is hoped that the housing officer will show a commitment to such a relationship in order to understand better the special housing needs of an individual experiencing severe mental distress.

The ongoing function of housing management should pay particular attention to the relationship between housing and mental health outlined earlier in this chapter. Continuous monitoring should be made of the tenant–landlord relationship, security of tenure, flexibility of rent payments, the potential need for the client to return to Hospital for a short stay, housing benefits, maintenance of the property, the need for housing transfers, the case for preferential treatment (and the client's potential refusal of preferential treatment because of the stigmatizing effects) and the potential need to be more available for case conferences or reviews on a regular basis. (Etherington, 1983).

As the potentially most frequent visitor to the client's home, the case manager should be aware of the functions involved in housing management. The role can occasionally be further extended to negotiating for clearance and cleaning (by the council 'dirty squad'); repair and redecorating; refurnishing, through helping the client to use or seek out special finance; accompanying the client to choose new household items; advocating with service utilities over the methods of payments or managing debts; putting up curtains and light bulbs; and finding the nearest shops. The Community Psychiatric Research Unit in Hackney has highlighted the need to supplement the informal support of friends and neighbours and that of other traditional psychiatric services, but not necessarily to take over all support to the point where the client is left totally dependent (Lovett, 1985).

The areas in which support may be required are potentially limitless but should not be assumed by the worker. They should arise out of the regular visiting and negotiating at the instigation of the client. In housing matters, as in many other issues, the case manager needs to be flexible and imaginative in response to the demands of the ongoing functions of support. So many, apparently small but actually large, daily requirements may go unnoticed or simply not taken on if workers are to adhere strictly to the limitations defined by professional status alone. The case manager will also be required to act as referral agent for other required services, such as home help, meals-on-wheels and district nursing, in order to support the clients' continuing residence in a property of their choice rather than being required to move to more highly supported accommodation.

When combined with the wider range of support services – through the needs arising in finance, occupation, health and self-care – the case manager may be in a better position to offer relevant services to the many people managed at home over many years, often with family members but without much contact with formal psychiatric services.

User initiatives

Initiated in the USA but still very limited in the UK, user groups have demonstrated supportive ordinary housing through their own projects. Chamberlin (1988) outlines the earlier work of the Mental Patients Association in setting up co-operative residences. These are shared houses run on entirely democratic lines by electing house co-ordinators to act as a supportive resource to all residents. The needed support, skills and management functions are discussed in regular house meetings, the philosophy being that everyone experiences difficulties in one form or another and these can be best managed by supporting each other. The wider development of the user initiatives has been impeded more by the obstacles presented by the system – particularly poor priorities for adequate funding and suitable property – rather than through the difficulties experienced by the users themselves.

Crisis houses

A useful adjunct to the wide range of housing support services that may be offered to clients in their own home is the availability of suitable short-stay crisis accommodation. Ideally, this should be in the form of ordinary housing (house, flats or bedsits) with access varying from a few days up to a few months. Such accommodation may be able to meet a wide variety of needs: crisis support, by removing vulnerable individuals from intolerable stresses associated with their own accommodation; temporary accommodation while their own home is undergoing necessary repairs or while awaiting a housing transfer; to promote discharge from a hospital bed before suitable accommodation has been allocated. Such a facility should ideally be seen as a supported placement, a preferable option to hospitalization, when the experience of distress is becoming too great. It may also be used as a form of assessment for people wishing to experience more independent living before they decide to apply for their own accommodation.

Whatever function this short-stay accommodation fulfils, it is vitally important to assess the relevant needs for supporting the individuals during their stay. Whoever manages the crisis accommodation should not be left with all the responsibilities for support, e.g. a voluntary sector owned flat or house, should be offered the support necessary from the statutory sector specialist services. Again, the functions of housing management and personal support may need to be clearly delineated.

SUMMARY

The House of Commons Social Services Committee (1985) reported that the provision and co-ordination of community residential options was clearly inadequate when compared with the pace of closure of the large mental hospitals. Many writers have wholeheartedly agreed with these conclusions throughout the much longer history of the movement towards a greater emphasis on community care (Ramon, 1988; Ryan, Ford and Clifford, 1991; Pilling, 1991).

Howat *et al.* (1988) suggest that a failure to integrate housing policy for people with special needs is the direct result of disjointed and poorly co-ordinated plans from the different service sectors. Pilling (1991) carries the argument further to suggest that the ultimate consequence of poorly conceived plans and a lack of co-ordination has been to contribute to, rather than reduce, the problem of homelessness among people with long-term severe mental illness.

A plethora of organizational responses has developed over the last forty years to meet the residential needs of this client group in the community (Wing and Morris, 1981; Lavender and Holloway, 1988; Pilling, 1991). More recently, the steadily growing concern is to meet the clients' preferred option for ordinary housing with flexible degrees of support to reflect the fluctuating levels of need over time (Heginbotham, 1985a; McAusland, 1985).

While there will always be a need for some provision of more highly structured and supported accommodation in the form of hostels and nursing homes (Pilling, 1991), Garety (1988) argues that the overriding principle of housing policy should be that of 'choice' over 'placement'. A case management response as advocated by Onyett (1992) could facilitate the provision of flexible levels of support to a client's own home as a more preferable response to one that would require the client to change accommodation in order to achieve different levels of support.

Such methods of outreach case management are also being advocated in services for the homeless mentally ill population (Bachrach and Nadelson, 1988; Brent-Smith and Dean, 1990). Timms and Fry (1989) argue that such approaches would be better targeted towards the services that have traditionally been used by homeless populations, rather than necessarily encouraging the take-up of existing psychiatric out-patient services.

6

Finance

FUNDING COMMUNITY MENTAL HEALTH SERVICES

Successive governments have produced policy statements proposing that the community care initiatives should improve services for the priority care client groups, but the authorities empowered to implement these policies are frequently left complaining that the funding levels to set up the new services are quite simply not sufficient (Mahoney, 1988).

Some of the expenditure figures have been indicated in the introductory chapter. But even with government claims about increasing expenditure in total figures, the costs of new treatments and medical advances have demanded considerable expenditure, with the result that mental health services receive a decreased proportion of total health service expenditure. Yet, the extent of change required by a move from institutional to community-based care requires a large capital expenditure to set up the new facilities, as well as a large expenditure to ensure the training and retraining of staff to perform the tasks appropriate to a new style of service. It is difficult to envisage just how these significant changes can be accommodated in a reducing proportion of total health service expenditure.

The difficulties are further compounded when we look at expenditure on mental health services by the local authorities. They are currently being required by central government policy to accept increasing responsibility for the co-ordination and provision of social and health aspects of community care. The overall spending by local authorities on mental health services is reported to be in single percentage figures (less than 5%), subject to wide local variations, but generally seen as a lower priority than spending on child care, the elderly and learning difficulties client groups. This, in turn, is having a knock-on effect on the voluntary sector which finds itself in more competitive circumstances when seeking out grant aid and funding from local authority sources. Local authorities are more frequently finding their own sources of funding from central government either being 'capped' in total or carrying specific restrictions and guidelines for different aspects of their finances.

In recent years, the expectation of central government is that a significant proportion of funding for new community facilities will come from the releasing of capital from the large psychiatric hospitals targeted for closure. The difficulty with such an expectation has been the time delay between the early need for capital finance to set up the new facilities and the later availability of the finance released by a closure of a hospital. In reality, a long-stay hospital has to greatly reduce the total number of residents before it can begin to release the capital. The necessary bridging loans from central finance to cover the short-term double expenditure by district health authorities have not been easily forthcoming.

The 'dowry' system of releasing health authority money with individual patients discharged to the community has also proved to be inadequate in terms of funding the wide range of necessary community services. Generally, this source of money is too narrowly targeted, accompanied by too many restrictions on its use and felt to be too low to meet the range of community needs (Mahoney, 1988).

Over the past 15 years a number of different funding schemes have been introduced by central government to encourage the development of community services. The difficulty appears to continue to lie in the small-scale 'tinkering' with projects rather than establishing a comprehensive system of national financing of community care. 'Joint finance' was introduced in 1976 to encourage partnership developments between health and local authorities; this initiative helped establish a number of small individual projects but failed to meet any grander objectives. This was largely because local authorities were unable to consider committing themselves to the longer-term funding implications for large numbers of community projects.

Further individual projects have been established through inner-city partnership, urban aid, health authority support of housing associations and more recently the mental illness specific grant. But each has failed to initiate a more consolidated approach to the funding of community care. Charitable trusts have occasionally provided the start-up capital funding for individual projects, and social security funding has been targeted to cover some of the housing costs.

The House of Commons Social Services Committee 1985 drew attention to the shortfall of health authority spending on the development of community services and indicated a need for central funding over a number of years to address the problem adequately. The Kings Fund College (1987) extended the proposal by suggesting the setting up of a national budget for community care, with the co-ordination of all developments to be addressed by a government community care and expenditure review group. So far, the political will has not matched the rhetoric from any political party, and the widespread *ad hoc* system of funding individual projects from different sources continues.

PERSONAL FINANCE

The need for adequate personal finance is one of the essential components for living in the community, yet the difficulties of trying to gain paid employment leaves the majority of people who experience severe mental distress surviving on a minimum subsistence level provided through the system of social security payments. Living on social security benefits means having to be very careful in accounting for every penny spent; it means having to deal with a large and confusing government department; and it can mean many hours spent queuing and waiting in quite degrading, and sometimes intimidating, social security offices (Davis, 1985; Shamash, 1991).

In this chapter, I propose to look at the options available for maintaining the necessary basic income to survive in what often amounts to no more than a poverty trap. Resorting to survival skills also becomes compounded by the disadvantages associated with a recurring illness or disability. My difficulty is one of presenting the complex financial arrangements in a general but understandable way, without necessarily focusing on the finer details of individual benefits which are constantly changing. The details of these benefits are far better documented in the specialist reference books, such as those published by the Child Poverty Action group (Lakhani and Read, 1990; Rowland, 1990).

Meteyard (1990) suggests that the various welfare benefit entitlements are constantly changing for a number of reasons, primarily 'the lessening or worsening conditions or circumstances to which some benefits may be linked; the periodic changes of emphasis of governments which change the system of rates and eligibility; and the fluctuations of local costs and entitlements such as rents, travel allowances, charitable grants, and so on.' The frequency of such changes seems to be more an arbitrary factor of political will rather than a response to the needs of the service users; the latter having to frequently rely on the hope of advice from knowledgeable support workers, or conversely remain ignorant of their full entitlements.

A further dilemma of this chapter is the need to indicate ways in which people experiencing severe mental distress can supplement their basic benefit incomes, but without prescribing budgeting strategies which will superficially condone the poverty endemic in the system. We all need to help our clients make ends meet, but we have a responsibility to advocate for more rather than reinforcing the insufficiency of the current system.

The basic level of benefit, is according to social security legislation, meant to cover all the basic living expenses, such as food; fuel; buying, cleaning, repairing and replacing clothing and shoes; travel; laundry costs; toiletries; cleaning materials; replacement of small household goods, such as light bulbs and crockery; leisure and amenity items such as TV and radio, newspapers, alcohol and tobacco (Davis, 1985). Supplementary additions are available for some aspects of illness and disability, but the reality for many people is still one of reducing the consumption of one necessity to accommodate a small amount of another or, in other words, eating less in order to afford heating for a short period of time. The individual is often required by circumstances to learn some 'real' life skills never addressed in rehabilitation programmes – such as patching old shoes with newspapers to prolong their life. Living on social security benefits in the 1990s can necessitate the development of an acute survival instinct.

The scope for 'advocacy' work appears to be enormous in the area of personal finances but, all too often, the support services either find themselves barely able to keep pace with the changes to the system or to continue with a professional blindness to the reality of poverty. In the latter case, ideas of improving the quality of environment, improving social interaction or improving the adequacy of diet are frequently put forward as goals for successful community rehabilitation without real consideration for the financial costs of these measures.

Davis (1985) recommends that the immediate practical steps for professionals should be to check that each individual (and family) is receiving the maximum benefits they are entitled to, to address the need to talk about financial worries and to work to influence positive change in the system through its policies. These requirements also involve knowing the limitations of your own knowledge, knowing where to expand your knowledge and knowing who else to contact for expert advice –including welfare rights experts, Citizens' Advice Bureaux, social security offices and information leaflets.

SOURCES OF PERSONAL INCOME

Before addressing the system of social security benefits and other sources of financial support for individual people, I propose to outline the individual circumstances of two particular individuals. These illustrations will help to indicate the wide range of financial circumstances that a case manager may be called upon to address. Furthermore, they should also give a focus to our attention on interventions outlined later in this chapter.

PERSONAL PROFILE

Joseph is a 32-year-old single man, born in Kenya following his parents' migration from Goa. His parents, an elder sister and two brothers live in Kenya, while his younger sister migrated to London a year after Joseph.

Joseph moved to London in 1983 with the intention of furthering his education with computer training, but his sister also implies that the decision was partly taken to escape from his parents' growing concern about his mental condition and neglectful behaviour. In Kenya Joseph had achieved two 0-levels through a further education college; he undertook a short course in electrical repairs and had a brief spell working in his brother's jewellery business. On arriving in London, his education and work record has tended to follow a chequered pattern, working for varying amounts of time in a fast-food restaurant, on a government training scheme, labouring and working as a kitchen porter. The latter job lasted for over 12 months, with Joseph inexplicably stopping work at a time when the employer considered his work record to be good.

The pattern of accommodation has followed a similar chaotic pattern, with his first few years in London being spent in a number of hostels without showing any signs of settling in one place. His sister agreed to share a two-bedroom council flat, on the basis that he may not be able to manage a tenancy by himself. This arrangement has continued for nearly five years, but the relationship is very poor and both of them wish to seek separate accommodation for different reasons – Joseph feels his sister interferes too much in his life and his sister occasionally feels threatened by him, but continues to be concerned by his apparent inability to cope without some support and supervision.

Joseph now has a steadily growing psychiatric and forensic history. His first admission to a psychiatric hospital was in 1980 in Kenya, at the age of 21. His parents had been influential in requesting an assessment and admission. He remained in hospital for one month. He was reported to have regained some of his interests after treatment but received no follow-up services after his discharge. After arriving in London, Joseph has displayed a progressive deterioration in his own personal care, a number of criminal offences and two further hospital admissions linked to his arrests in 1985 and 1991. In psychiatric terms, he is considered to be suffering from a schizophrenic illness, displaying more of the negative features of neglect and social withdrawal. He has been described as displaying an 'emotional refrigeration', with very few affective responses to the approaches of other people.

The forensic history has consisted of assault in 1983, criminal damage in 1985 and 1989, theft and a further charge of assault causing actual bodily harm in 1990 and the non-payment of court costs in 1991 (for an earlier offence). Some of these offences are closely linked to the chaotic pattern of financial responsibilities adopted by Joseph.

His income has come solely from social security benefits since giving up his job as a kitchen porter, but his pattern of spending tends to be quite irresponsible and beyond his personal means of income. In general, Joseph spends his money on inexplicable train journeys to other cities in the UK, food, alcohol and tobacco. He has managed to attempt to extend his purchasing ability through ordering many goods by setting up accounts with mail order companies, but he only repays a small fraction of the bills he accumulates on these accounts. As a result of the ease with which he is able to set up these accounts, Joseph now finds himself facing a number of threats of court action from the different companies for non-payment of goods received. His financial circumstances are made more chaotic through his intermittent payments of rent and outstanding court costs and non-payment of poll tax to the local council.

The characteristic of chaos extends to many other aspects of Joseph's life, not just his finances. His ideas for daytime activity can shift from full-time employment to full-time education, to day-centre attendance, to the take-up of wide-ranging sports and recreation activities, all in successive sentences. But reality contradicts all of these perceptions as he follows very little actual structure, has no set destinations when he does go out of the flat, is quite variable in his meeting of appointments and tends to limit his social interactions to children in the same flats or the adjacent school (bringing further concerns and threats from local parents and residents). His care of his part of the flat also reflects the self-neglect evident in his usually dishevelled appearance; water taps or the cooker may occasionally be left unattended and he occasionally leaves the front door to the flat open, inviting theft.

Positive characteristics

- He will occasionally maintain his wide interest in reading.
- He retains a single-minded attitude towards increasing his spending ability (though not always by legal means).
- He has an intermittent but fairly recent work history with a potentially reasonable work reference.
- He has continued concern and support from his sister.

Joseph's own statement of needs:

- a full-time job to stimulate his interests and provide a better income;
- to return to a suitable and supportive hostel that will offer both accommodation and the option to socialize;
- to join a local sports centre to develop an active interest in sport.

CASE STUDY

Moving from financial crisis to financial crisis

Edwin is a 60-year-old man, profiled in more detail in Chapter 4. Since their marriage in 1989, Edwin and his wife have received a joint Invalidity Benefit weekly payment from social security but no other source of income. One of the main focuses of the work with this couple has been on assessing their financial entitlements and supporting them through successive financial crises as they arise.

A part of the problem has been paranoid feelings of persecution experienced by Edwin on a long-term basis including the strongly held belief that he is being denied extra state benefits, a pools win and payments on a lapsed insurance policy, because all organizations and authorities are conspiring against him. This situation has necessitated much investigative work by the case manager so that Edwin can be presented with clear facts about individual circumstances rather than have his claims instantly denied as being the product of a paranoid disposition.

The plan to assess and increase their income seemed most feasible, on the grounds of his wife's physical incapacity, through an application for mobility allowance. The first potential crisis arose through rent account statements indicating moderate rent arrears on Edwin's previous council tenancy and large arrears, in excess of £1000, on his current tenancy. The investigations of the case manager prompted the local housing department to acknowledge that nearly all of this problem arose from unclaimed housing benefit, because a previous hospital admission had not been notified to the council, and because Edwin had failed to receive advice about his entitlements during a previous period of time when he was receiving no formally nominated source of support. In this situation, the case manager had a dual educative role – to inform the client of the full entitlements and to inform the housing authority of the problems arising out of difficult personal circumstances and the experience of severe mental distress.

No sooner had the first financial crisis settled then the couple received an extremely large quarterly telephone bill (over £800), with demands for immediate payment or risk losing their telephone and facing further court actions. Edwin and his wife have a strong need for a telephone on health grounds but make very few outgoing calls. Further investigations made by the case manager to British Telecom resulted in confirmation of the accuracy of the bill with an itemized print out listing each call made, but it was a third party abusing the use of their telephone. Following subsequent negotiations, they were requested to pay off £60 a month from the debt and to accept a technical bar on the telephone blocking any further outgoing calls.

A further financial crisis was brought on by the late, but sudden, council decision to offer Edwin and his wife a housing transfer to a flat more suitable for his wife's physical disablities. In order to help them to fund such a move, an application had to be made for a social security grant or loan, involving help with telephone calls, completion of detailed forms, support at the social security interview and some advice on priority spending for new furniture.

THE SOCIAL SECURITY SYSTEM

For the vast majority of people experiencing long-term severe mental distress the social security system will be their only source of income, yet, despite their health difficulties and generally impoverished personal circumstances, the individual client (and for that matter the community support worker) is faced with a most complex and baffling system of procedures and form-filling, of interviews and waiting, of prioritizing and disappointment and, in some circumstances, of degradation and despair. Such are the complexities and sources of disappointment that a deep psychological barrier to access is set up for many clients resulting in under-claiming of entitlements, lack of knowledge of entitlements and anger with the system.

Not only are the individual benefits constantly being reviewed and changed, even the organization's name has seemed to undergo several recent changes – from the Department of Health and Social Security (DHSS) to the Department of Social Security (DSS) and then to the Benefits Agency (BA). The changes in name cannot disguise what for many people has proved to be an extremely dehumanizing experience.

For the majority of social security claimants the system consists of confusing forms, a wait in a queue to sign your continued status of unemployment and a further wait at home for the giro payment to arrive. For the few, considered to be 'problem cases' (which include many people in the long-term mentally ill client group), the office system of repetitive interviews, long waits and counter payments exists. Shamash (1991) sadly, but fairly accurately, portrays a picture of inner-city offices: 'Each social security office is a place of seething resentment – a rare sort of hell, compounded of noise, poverty, filth, despair and utter frustration.'

The all too frequent situation is one of toughened glass screens separating the necessarily anonymous and over-stressed officers, presenting the inflexible face of a complex system, from the dishevelled and poverty-stricken lives of claimants exhausted by the stresses of having to survive on minimal sums of money and waiting their turn for hours amidst the frequent expressions of anger from frustrated fellow-claimants.

The office can be a place of heightened confrontation where claimants often believe that officers deliberately lie to add to their personal misery – 'the files are in another part of the office', 'the giro is in the post', 'the computer in Glasgow (or Newcastle or Belfast) is processing the necessary information before payment can be authorized' are all met with a stream of abusive retorts. The result of such working conditions tends to be very high staff turnover, stress-related illness and a high risk of personal attack (Shamash, 1991).

Whilst the above description appears bleak in the extreme, it nonetheless occurs repeatedly and is the reality that clients may have to experience in order to pursue their own claims for specific benefits. It also provides a clear explanation of why so many entitlements can go unclaimed by people in this client group.

Categories of social security benefit

Essentially, benefit entitlements are divided into those which are 'means-tested' and those that are 'non-means-tested', though further subdivisions render the system far more complex even before one begins to look at the criteria for qualification associated with individual benefits.

Means-tested benefits are entitlements that ensure an income does not fall below what the government thinks an individual or family need. They act as a 'top-up' for any other income a client may be receiving (including topping up other benefits). But the amount received is determined by 'testing' for appropriate qualification criteria; the size of a family and the amount of income received from any other sources. Some means-tested benefits are designed to pay for specific charges or costs, e.g. towards the payment of rent.

The main benefits in this category (at February 1992) are Income Support, Family Credit, Housing Benefit, Community Charge Benefit, the Social Fund (described later in this chapter), health benefits and education benefits. Most non-means-tested benefits count as income when calculating an entitlement to a means-tested benefit, the exception being Attendance Allowance and Mobility Allowance (both replaced by Disability Living Allowance in April 1992). The result often means that the entitlement is reduced, or even lost completely, by the other income received (Lakhani and Read, 1990).

The category of non-means-tested benefits is designed to provide a basic weekly income instead of earnings and entitlement depends on meeting specific criteria rather than an investigation of personal financial affairs. Many of these benefits exist to compensate for an inability to work, whether through unemployment, sickness, pregnancy or old age; and some exist to meet specific needs arising from disability or child care, irrespective of ability to work (Rowland, 1990).

The non-means-tested benefits may be categorized in a number of different ways, but the most frequently used subdivisions are those of:

1. contributory benefits: unemployment benefit, sickness benefit, invalidity benefit and widow's pension – these are paid out of the National Insurance Fund derived from contributions paid in by employers, employees, the self-employed and some voluntary contributions;
2. non-contributory benefits: severe disablement allowance, invalid care allowance, attendance allowance (some change to Disability Living Allowance in April 1992) and benefits in respect of children – these are paid out of general taxation.

The benefits generally paid in respect of periods of incapacity to work require their eligibility to be covered by medical certificates, renewable for varying periods of time – usually 3, 6 or 12 months. But the new non-means-tested benefits being introduced in April 1992, namely Disability Living Allowance and Disability Working Allowance, will also attempt to shift the emphasis from the medical assessment required for the previous Attendance Allowance and Mobility Allowance to self-assessment through answering questions only on the form. The new system will employ independent adjudication officers to calculate entitlements by checking the answers written down against certain qualifying criteria. This change will again highlight the need for the individual applicant to seek out good advice and help when completing the form – which should be available, directly or indirectly, through the case manager.

The case manager should be prepared to assess all available means for maximizing a client's entitlement but, generally,

non-means-tested benefits provide a passport to other entitlements as well as requiring less frequent reapplication and proof
of circumstances.

Disagreement with the benefits decisions

The most common option is to follow a specific line of appeal.
In the case of some benefits, this will involve a further decision
by a tribunal. The new allowances mentioned above will be
overseen by an appeals tribunal, chaired by a lawyer and
including representatives to give a medical opinion, someone
with experience of disability, someone of the same sex as the
claimant, someone to put the social security department's view
and a tribunal clerk. The claimant will have the right to be
accompanied by a friend and/or an adviser.

Other avenues for appeal may be through a local MP to the
Secretary of State or Minister for Social Security or to a local
ombudsman in the case of appeals against local council
decisions.

It is important to note that the area of finances is strongly
determined by an emphasis on problems in order to promote
the entitlements of the individual. This can conflict with other
philosophies of working, particularly the approach of the
strengths model of case management. This apparent contradiction needs to be assimilated by the worker to ensure the
possibility of best outcomes for the client.

The social fund

A special reference is made to this aspect of the system because
it differs fundamentally from most other benefits mentioned
above. The Social Fund is a system of loans and community
care grants introduced in 1988 to replace the previous 'single
payments'. It differs from other current benefits in that it is
particularly targeted to meet some of the needs associated with
community care. It is particularly meant to help with the costs
of staying in, or returning to, the community rather than an
institution, and to cover items such as essential furniture,
repairs, moves to more suitable accommodation and other
exceptional pressures on claimants and their families.

The case manager should have knowledge of the Social
Fund as a method of financing special circumstances for the

individual client. But there has been widespread criticism of the system from its inception – largely against its prime function of reducing some social security costs by its strict criteria for entitlements, cash limits imposed on individual social security offices, the emphasis on using loans over and above grants and the high rate of loan refusals on the grounds that claimants will not be able to afford the repayments.

Meteyard (1990) suggests that it would be quite anomalous to envisage Social Fund loans as 'assistance', because they put the recipient into debt with an immediate lowering of their weekly benefit income. He argues that the community worker has a responsibility to help the client, where possible, find other alternatives which may not incur so much debt and with reduced levels of repayment. Where clients are not eligible for the Social Fund (because they are not in receipt of Income Support), they may apply for a social security 'crisis loan', which again incurs the same potential for debt and repayment but still provides an option for covering the immediate costs at a time of crisis.

'Urgent case payments' are a further option to be considered, under circumstances where hardship is likely to be experienced from forces beyond the claimant's control. The most frequent situation in which these payments are made is a possible delay in receiving other benefits to which the client is entitled, such as a delay in sending out a pension book renewal. The payment is normally made in the form of a giro, over the social security office counter, for up to 90% of the normal weekly entitlement.

Much of the information in this section on social security benefits is subject to frequent changes. The above information should only be taken as a guide, with more up-dated information being available in written guidance leaflets from the 'Benefits Agency' or annual publications e.g. the 'Child Poverty Action Group'.

Methods of payment

As mentioned above, the normal weekly benefit payments are either made through a weekly giro sent to a home address in the post, weekly giros paid over a social security counter in particular circumstances, or a pension book for up to 13 weeks which is cashed on a weekly basis at a nominated post office.

In certain circumstances an individual's money may be controlled by another agency in law, through court of protection or an appointee. These regulations are currently referred through social workers rather than a generic case manager.

Unforeseen difficulties can occasionally arise for a client if a large sum is backdated or a one off payment is made through the Social Fund which is in excess of the amount a post office is prepared to cash (currently £250). These payments are also often made through a girobank order, requiring clearance through a bank account. Such circumstances do little to relieve the initial crisis necessitating the claim if the claimant is then unable to make immediate use of the money. The social security office can be requested to split such payments between redeemable giros in order to meet the needs of the immediate crisis.(NB: Most social security payments must be reduced, by law, when a claimant has been admitted to hospital for more than six weeks. This is to reflect the meeting of certain 'board and lodging' needs by the hospital during the admission).

Besides the direct receipt of different forms of income, a creative mind and a thorough knowledge of local community resources may enable people to cut a few financial corners or to budget limited resources more economically.

Davis (1985) suggests that

> hospital and community-based services for people recovering from mental illness can provide material benefits: a good, low-cost, hot lunch; washing and drying facilities; access to second-hand clothing; cookers, so that people can prepare a good meal to take home; hairdressing; opportunities to make clothes or knit. Facilities like these can mean a great deal to people managing on a low income, and can contribute as much, if not more, to their sense of well-being and confidence as any therapeutic group.

Knowledge of the local area should go well beyond the services exclusively used by people experiencing severe long-term mental distress to include other outlets for cheap and/or second-hand goods, cheap nutritious meals and furniture from local council or voluntary sector storage as well as private sector shops. Applications may be made for charitable funding and grants or gifts for specific goods, such as items of furniture or televisions and other electrical goods. Travel permit applications, if successful, can dissolve nearly all expected travelling costs.

In terms of budgeting, a client can be advised to seek out the many arrangements now available from organizations – standing order payments, spreading payments wider than just the quarterly bills, use of budget stamps to save towards bills, meters or rechargeable key schemes to manage consumption of electricity, coin-operated telephones or bar systems to reduce telephone use and applications for discounts, rebates or exemptions from specific payments. Some bills may be able to be paid by direct deductions of social security benefits at source.

The case manager may be involved in negotiating debt agreements or occasional writing-off of the debt, through making out 'exceptional case' circumstances. (NB: A debt written-off should not allow a client to raise unrealistic expectations that they can continue to ignore basic financial constraints in the hope that the case manager will arrange for future debts to be written-off – as was the case with Joseph in this chapter's personal profile.)

In small, isolated cases, a mental health team's funds may be partially set up to cover certain 'rehabilitation' costs. Creative use of such funds may enable small crisis loans, in addition to the payment for materials, equipment or food considered a necessary part of rehabilitation work.

ROLES FOR THE CASE MANAGER

The area of finance, like so many others, tends to throw up a diversity of functions for the case manager to perform, but it also, arguably, produces more controversy around who ideally should be performing the function of welfare rights adviser.

One function is that of offering knowledge and advice, even in an educative role, to the client. The case manager may also act as a filter by referring or directing clients to more expert sources of advice. He or she is also likely to be called upon to do more advocacy work in the area of finance than any other area, through negotiating agreements and debt write-offs to writing letters of support of their situation, and through acting as a support when required to accompany a client to an appointment or interview. With an additional need to help with the process of claiming benefits, rebates and exemptions, this area of work requires a great deal of telephone and written responses.

In response to the question of who should ideally be carrying out the bulk of the financial assessments and support work, there are a number of options:

- welfare rights advisers;
- social workers;
- user/independent advocacy groups;
- individual in team with special interest (regardless of qualification);
- all team members for own clients (regardless of qualifications).

There are no special right or wrong answers: the only option truly set up for this specialist purpose is the welfare rights adviser; the others are likely to engage in multiple roles. Though the social worker is often regarded by the other professionals as holding the specific expertise, social workers do not necessarily see themselves limited to this specialism, and would be the first to agree that it needs regular attention to keep pace with the social security changes that constantly take place. The user/independent advocacy groups would claim an independent objectivity not possessed by the professional workers.

In defence of keeping the role within the team, the specific keyworkers will know their clients' wants and needs better than outside agencies; they can combine a financial educative role with education in other areas, where necessary; and, as stated in Chapter 3, financial matters offer one of the best practical options for helping along the engagement process between client and support worker. It is advisable to have one team member develop a special interest in ongoing changes to the system, to act as a focal point for the knowledge of the team.

Whatever the arrangement, it is important to have the role of financial advice clearly accepted inside and outside the team. This is a specialist function and poor advice is more likely to result in legal action against the adviser in the growing climate of litigation. The new benefits being introduced in April 1992 may potentially increase the role of the case manager, particularly with the emphasis on self-assessments reducing the need for formal medical assessments.

SUMMARY

The funding of mental health services and the personal finances of individuals experiencing severe long-term distress both present circumstances of ongoing concern to the case manager working in community mental health. However, these two areas should be viewed separately when considering the mechanisms for providing adequate financial resources.

Beyond the verbal assurances of politicians to finance the new community health services, there is still no proper commitment to a central method of national co-ordination and funding (Kings Fund College, 1987). The release of capital from hospital closure programmes is generally timed too late to ensure continuity of replacement community resources, and other sources of funding tend to exist through *ad hoc* schemes and arrangements, none of which could remotely be seen to underpin the real resource implications of an adequate provision of community care services (Mahoney, 1988).

A distinct poverty trap is set up for people experiencing the long-term consequences of severe mental distress (Davis, 1985). Employment opportunities seem extremely limited, leaving individuals to depend largely on the basic subsistence levels offered through social security benefits. This system is in itself extremely complex and somewhat bewildering to the individual experiencing severe distress. Client advocates, including case managers, need regular access to accurate and up-to-date information on the system of benefit entitlements, rates, exemptions and rebates. Some benefits will open entitlement to others, while some result in an exclusion from others (Lakhani and Read, 1990; Rowland, 1990).

The case manager can assume a wide range of roles in relation to the financial circumstances of individual clients. Knowledge of the benfits system is vital, but also knowing your own limitations and who to refer on to for further expert advice is equally important. Advocacy roles may well become the primary focus of intervention. Appropriate support may also require knowledge of other opportunities in the local community for indirectly influencing an individual's income – budgeting schemes, bargains and discounts, or free access to services such as a washing machine in a local day centre (Davis, 1985).

7

Activities of daily living

DEFINITION

For most of the profession's history, occupational therapy has shown a significant concern for independent functioning abilities through the activities of daily living. Yet, despite the frequent claims of this interest as a 'core' skill, there is still no universally accepted definition of the concepts involved. This may be attributed, in part, to the wide range of elements covered by the title, but it is now increasingly being acknowledged by occupational therapists that there is a need to define, standardize and measure activities of daily living more precisely (Murdock, 1992).

There appears to be broad agreement, in the literature, about the range of functions that may be included under the term ADL, but valid and reliable research remains patchy (Eakin, 1989a; 1989b). Furthermore, within the material published by occupational therapists, the emphasis relates more to work undertaken in the fields of physical medicine and the care of the elderly with very little space devoted to the subject in the psychiatric literature.

Reed (1984) and Hopson (1987) discuss a range of assumptions underpinning the need to address activities of daily living. These relate to the need: (a) for baseline measures of competence, (b) to guide the encouragement of change, (c) to compare optimum and maximum levels of skill and (d) to understand the factors which influence competence. The consensus of opinion suggests that the 'activities' include all of the day-to-day functions which most of us take for granted as being a part of our daily routines, and in which a failure to perform would suddenly render us significantly more dependent on others.

It is a much wider concept than that of self-care alone. As Willson (1987) suggests, the adequate performance of such a range of activities requires more than just the necessary cognitive and physical abilities – it requires a sense of personal identity and awareness of the responses of others; it involves a desire to achieve a degree of physical comfort which motivates the desire for self-care; and it involves the achievement of a degree of autonomy which promotes feelings of independence and personal control.

In simple terms, activities of daily living would include the personal skills of caring for self and the immediate environment, and the wider personal and social skills necessary to perform a multitude of interactions with other people.

The range of activities of daily living includes:

- personal appearance and hygiene – including washing, bathing; care of hair, nails, teeth; cleaning and repair of clothing and footwear;
- domestic skills – including shopping, cooking, diet and nutrition;
- household management – including dusting, vacuuming, refuse disposal and minor electrical replacements;
- family and child care – including education, play and safety;
- family planning and sexual matters – including sexuality, sex education, contraception and counselling needs;
- budgeting and personal administration – including balancing income and expenditure, form-filing, post, entitlements and personal rights to peace and safety;
- conversational and social skills – including verbal and non-verbal behaviour;
- mobility and transfers – include physical abilities or disabilities, accessibility and entitlements;
- leisure, education, training and work activities (addressed in Chapter 8).

Activity analysis

The breadth of meaning applied to the term 'activity' is illustrated thus by Trombly (1989):

Activity of many kinds define human existence. Activities are inherently important to the individual not only to fulfil basic needs and wants but also to achieve mastery and competence. Activity is the treatment occupational therapy offers to patients based on the hypothesis that activities can produce change away from dysfunctional and toward functional behaviour. ... The use of purposeful activity makes treatment meaningful to the client and makes him his own co-therapist.

If we agree that a unique characteristic of occupational therapy is the use of carefully planned activity as a treatment medium, then the method used for planning is that of activity analysis – a process of closely examining activities to determine their component parts; to describe, structure and evaluate the components in the detail required to ensure that the appropriate activity can be matched to the functional and personal needs of the individual.

Willson (1984) suggests that the component parts of an activity can be evaluated in terms of environmental requirements, time for completion, scope for modification and the complexity of the skills required. Furthermore, tasks should be evaluated in terms of their range of demands: interpersonal/social, independence/dependence, cognitive, physical and emotional.

Professional responsibilities

Addressing the requirements for personal care skills is often seen as a shared responsibility between the nursing and occupational therapy professions. In general terms, the nursing profession is concerned with aspects of an individual's self-care, particularly personal appearance and hygiene, family planning and sexual matters whereas the occupational therapy profession stakes its claim to the core skill of applying activity analysis to a fuller range of functional activity.

Brown (1991) questioned occupational therapists, community psychiatric nurses and social workers about their views on the functions of occupational therapy. One of the responses was a shared recognition of the OT role in its use of activity as therapeutic intervention to involve and motivate the client, but there was also an understanding of the occupational therapist's unique ability to teach practical life skills and coping strategies using everyday situations as a treatment medium.

A unique role assumed by a case management approach to community support, is that of widely assessing and assisting people in ADL in their own environments. All aspects of a person's ADL are seen as a vital priority for support, often requiring the case manager to offer the choice of much more collaborative practical involvement than would be the case with most traditional professional services in the community. The quality of those inputs may also be distinguished by their intrinsic acknowledgement of the client's individual approaches to, and eccentricities in, problem-solving, while offering basic practical alternatives as a matter of choice.

THEORY AND PRACTICE

Definitions, models and complex analyses belong to the world defined by professionals where there is a requirement to show how knowledge specifically relates to a body of theory, and where competition for recognition and clear identity requires a profession to demonstrate how its claims are composed and can be measured.

The realities of activities of daily living, as personally experienced by an individual, do not share the same cold and clinical characterisitcs of the professional assessment and skills training programmes. The following personal profile and case study are included at this point in the chapter, to give specific examples of how the functions of activities of daily living may be experienced, and occasionally addressed, in community settings. It is hoped that these examples may return us from pondering on the theoretical to a glimpse of the practical, and thus set the scene for subsequent consideration of how these functions may be approached in the reality of clients' lives and available creative community resources. Whilst these examples may initially evoke a somewhat bleak and negative picture of neglect, they nevertheless serve to illustrate real circumstances and survival instincts which are not always acknowledged or addressed in the development of a skills training programme.

PERSONAL PROFILE

Bill if a 57-year-old man, born in England, who has lived in different areas of London throughout his life. His family have moved to different parts of England as well as Europe and North America, and he has had little or no contact with other family members since leaving home to serve his National Service 40 years ago.

Bill generally describes a life of unhappiness and loss which has ultimately rendered him a recluse in his council bedsit, with little desire to make contact with the outside world for anything other than the necessity of eating.

Following what he describes as an unhappy childhood, beaten by his father and bullied at school, the first, and possibly most psychologically damaging, loss came when he lost his leg as a result of being shot whilst doing National Service in the army out in Egypt. Regret at the decision to volunteer to go out to Egypt is still prominent in his mind some 38 years later.

The second damaging loss followed some 12 years later when his wife of 8 years took their 5-year-old son and left him, apparently as a result of no longer being able to manage his extremes of behaviour relating to mental health problems (this is Bill's own perception of the reasoning). He has had no contact with them, 26 years later on. This loss has also served to highlight the estrangement from the rest of his family – maintaining only infrequent contact with one of his brothers living close to London.

Bill's mental health problems began shortly after the loss of his leg. He was admitted to a London hospital in 1955 with a depressive illness. Since 1962 he has been admitted to hospitals on 12 occasions with apparent mental health problems – diagnoses have varied from schizophrenia (1962), psychotic depression (1968), inadequate psychopath (1974), personality disorder (1975) to chronic paranoid schizophrenia (1979). The one constant feature has been a depressive element to his presentation throughout, with a serious suicide attempt following the departure of his wife and child. Bill has received community psychiatric nurse involvement for 15 years and case management involvement for the last two years. He continues to receive fortnightly depot injections.

Occupation and housing have both followed a changing pattern, until he settled some 10 years ago. His occupational history is highlighted in Chapter 8, but has included earlier periods of employment in cabinet-making, briefcase assembly and as a lift attendant. This was followed by attendances at different local day-care services. In the last 10 years he has had no formal commitment to any form of occupational status, preferring to live a more reclusive existence at home.

Similarly, his housing status followed a changing pattern of flats, bedsits and hostels following the departure of his wife and son. He has now settled into the same council bedsit for the last 10 years and occasionally expresses the wish to live his remaining days in this place he regards as home.

In terms of activities of daily living, Bill has adopted a very minimalist reclusive lifestyle in the darkness of his bedsit, behind closed doors and curtains, with the flicker of a badly repaired television and an endless succession of cigarettes to break the time spent sitting or lying on his bed.

Attention to self-care and wider social skills is characterized by extreme neglect. Bill rarely washes, never bathes and tends to wear the same limited range of clothing until the condition and odour compel one of his few visitors to demand that he throws them away. The condition of his bed and immediate surroundings is treated with the same neglect – he will urinate in bed or in a bucket beside his bed if he doesn't wish to move to the bathroom. Many cigarette ends float in the urine-filled bucket beside his bed. The case manager has occasional successes, in terms of helping Bill to pay for a replacement mattress and some infrequent use of sheets and a mattress cover. In conjunction with the home help, the case manager is also able to periodically encourage Bill to dispose of badly soiled items, to launder a few and buy basic replacements.

Much of the remainder of his bedsit remains unused, musty and choking from the mixture of urine and cigarette smells, with severely discoloured walls and ceiling. He has only limited need for a kitchen since he has a daily routine of buying a meal in a local restaurant which allows him in during off-peak periods, fearful that his appearance and hygiene may put off other customers during peak meal times. He occasionally uses a mobile snack bar beneath a nearby railway station if the restaurant is closed. The only other regular purchase is cigarettes. The aim of case management is to work with Bill's own statements of need. A secondary aim is to work in the longer term to help him understand possible detrimental effects of the general neglect of his appearance, hygiene and surrounding environment. Regular discussions over many months have resulted in Bill requesting that improvements to the decor of his home should be investigated, and he has hinted at a willingness to help with some painting of his flat (with help from the case manager).

Financially, he receives a war disability pension and severe disablement allowance. Budgeting is aided by a home help who has known him for the last 10 years. She will collect his money and buy extra clothes, food or cleaning materials which may be needed in the bedsit for her to offer a cleaning service. He permits the case manager to check his mail and deal with any financial matters that arise over his benefits, rent payments or council levy for taxes.

Mobility is by the use of crutches, though he has used a prosthetic limb temporarily and now and again suggests that he may make use of another if it were provided. He has occasional falls in the street, where uneven paving presents dangers to anyone with reduced mobility. He has also been mugged in the street following the cashing of his benefits pension book. Bill has spontaneously asked the case manager to check the maintenance of his elbow crutches, and to help him to follow the process of applying for a new prosthetic limb.

Social skills are generally poor, in that his appearance and hygiene, eating and smoking habits tend to be offensive to others who do not know him. Conversation skills are minimal, partly through few opportunities to practice, and partly through suspicion of others built up over a long history of loss and threat to his person, inside as well as outside the home. The effort to make conversation with him is occasionally rewarded by some positive verbal and non-verbal responses. He can gradually build up some trust

in a few people, but will still retain control of the relationship through not opening his door at times when he doesn't
wish contact or wishes to communicate that a worker's
aims are not in tune with his own.

Bill no longer indicates a desire to consider deeper relationships, sexual or otherwise. He makes occasional
reference to a lady friend some six years ago, who briefly
entered into a serious relationship but discontinued contact
after six months. This provided a further source of regret
and loss, but reinforces his apparent disinterest with the
idea of searching for any other relationships.

Bill has infrequently visited the one or two public houses
that will serve him in the local area. He has also engaged
in discussions with his case manager about visits outside
his flat, actually completing two leisure trips with the case
manager in the past two years. He will also infrequently
make use of the free travel enabled by his local authority
travel permit.

Positive characteristics

- He has a strong survival instinct to manage a very
  minimal lifestyle.
- There is a warmth of personality that rewards people
  who persevere with contact beyond the initial prejudices
  against neglected appearance and hygiene.
- He shows an ability to communicate experiences of
  distress to the case manager in order that he may now
  use support before the need for hospital admission.
- He has a strong sense of personal control over his use
  of services and contact with people.

Bill's own expression of needs:

- the occasional company offered by trusted visitors to
  his bedsit;
- a desire to revisit a local cinema to rekindle his past
  interest in western movies;
- to remain in his current council bedsit for the rest of his
  life;
- occasional opportunities to express his loss and sadness
  about the incident causing the loss of his leg and the

departure of his wife and son (but not to engage in any formal counselling);

- to keep taking the injections to prevent having to be admitted to hospital again;
- to consider the possible use of a new prosthetic leg.

CASE STUDY 1

A conflict over priorities between the client and others

Mary's circumstances have already been profiled in the introductory chapter and more briefly in other chapters. But activities of daily living are highlighted as a significant issue, focusing attention on the potential conflict between a person's failure to acknowledge the priority of personal care in the face of society's higher value on appearance and hygiene.

Mary has clearly stated priorities in terms of doing what is necessary to remain home rather than be admitted to hospital, and for maintaining the security of tenure of her flat. She appears not to see care of herself or the condition of her flat as of any particular priority for meeting her own needs. On most occasions she denies that she has any ADL difficulties. This denial is upheld despite her increasingly dirty, dishevelled and hirsute appearance and reports of mounting rubbish and filth within parts of the flat.

For Mary, a long history of offers of help and skills training has had little effect on her actual capabilities or her acceptance of regular support to maintain publicly acceptable standards of self-care and household management. The question arises as to whether she is making informed choices, but the indication from actions in other aspects of her life would suggest that she is aware of her personal circumstances. It remains for all regular contacts with her to maintain a dialogue and assessment that her health, or environmental health standards, are not causing her any danger.

She will sometimes accept help from a distant relative, including help to tidy the flat and to shave her excessive facial hair which results from endocrine problems. Unfortunately, this relative can only visit occasionally. Though the case manager is denied access to provide similar support, the aim is to monitor the situation from brief doorstep encounters and through liaison with the district nurse and relative, both of whom have more successful access to the flat. Mary also accepts meals-on-wheels rather than risk the danger of using a cooker with her extrapyramidal tremor. So the case manager ultimately co-ordinates some of the input from other necessary services and has Mary's co-operation to pay her money on her behalf into the social services office for the meals-on-wheels.

The exercise is one of becoming creative in the offers of help and encouragement, either through brief conversation with Mary or more formal written methods. In the meantime, the worries expressed by other people about Mary's mental health and appearance need to be absorbed by the case manager and addressed by the counter-argument of individual rights.

On the unfortunate occasions when she has been in hospital, for physical as well as mental health problems, Mary agreed to the case manager having access to her money and her flat so that its safety could be supervised and necessary decoration and general refurbishment could take place, including organizing the clearance of many belongings and replacing clothing, furniture, bedding and carpets.

ADL ASSESSMENT

For the occupational therapist this aspect of assessment forms a core function of the work. Though other professionals may refer a person for a self-care assessment by an OT the occupational therapist will generally assume a wider definition of activities of daily living. They are often able to offer a wider range of service to the individual client than the referrer was able to make the client aware of.

For the majority of occupational therapists, this wide range of assessment and treatment opportunities arises out of the diversity of materials, equipment, environments and expertise available in the OT department.

The professional requirement for assessment to have a more technical appearance has resulted in greater research demands for demonstrable validity and reliability of measures. Murdock (1992) suggests that an ADL assessment can only be regarded as clinically useful if it, firstly, provides a baseline for treatment and evidence of the effectiveness of a treatment programme and, secondly, allows for comparison between patients and also a change in a patient's performance over a period of time. Such requirements place stricter demands on the simulated environments developed in occupational therapy programmes so that comparisons can be made with fewer doubts cast about changing environmental factors.

Psychologists and occupational therapists have become more attracted to the comparative features of a range of assessment scales and measures. Rosen, Hadzi-Pavlovic and Parker (1989) give a detailed outline of their Life Skills Profile, but also consider a wide range of scales developed in relation to activities of daily living, highlighting factors such as format, costs, acceptability and utility of the assessment tool itself. However, the development and use of specific measures must be influenced by the extensive range of function covered by ADL. Murdock (1992) argues that inclusion and exclusion of functions must be made clear in the definition of a measure but, ultimately, a range of separate measures should be used to cover the whole range from self-care to social skills.

Assessment in the community

As with many others areas of need, activities of daily living in community settings are much more controlled by the desires of the client than is the case with the more artificial settings of hospital department or wards. Such shift of power is necessary, and right, to uphold the dignity of the individual in his or her own environment. It also means that, in practical terms, the issues around the activities of daily living should be about offering advice and support to promote personal choice, rather than any notion of coercing a person to meet the standards and values of others. It becomes vital to ascertain what clients perceive to be their own strengths and weaknesses

so that the priorities for offering support can be matched
to these needs. Failure to do so will generally result in
little co-operation with any care plans the case manager
generates.

A further reason for assessment focusing in the individual's
personal standards is the external influences that may affect
those standards – particularly family, peer group and cultural
factors which can influence the activities of daily living.

The assessment of activities of daily living in a person's
home environment is a very real assessment which may form
a basis for interventions that can bring about meaningful and
lasting positive changes. The assessment and treatment
programmes in the simulated environments are often valuable
in terms of considering generalized skills, but all too often the
benefit of the simulated training does not translate to the home
situation. The person who learns to cook on an electric cooker
in the department may be returning home to no cooking
facilities and would have been better served by considering
other aspects of diet and nutrition outside of the home. A
further criticism is the misrepresentation promoted by group
sessions in the department; whilst it is admirable to promote
the social side of catering and dining, the person returning
to live at home is poorly served by developing skills of
shopping and cooking for four. It can be concluded, therefore,
that such assessments are better undertaken in the client's
more usual environment if we are to give priority to their own
experience of reality. But we must still respect that simulated
environments do have a limited educational value.

Methods of assessment

The methods used are very much the same as those outlined
by Willson (1984):

- discussion and observation of skills by the client;
- discussion with significant others – carers, friends and other
  staff;
- completing formal practical assessments, set up with the
  individual in his or her own home;
- completing written questionnaires, measures and assessment scales with the client.

By far the most important method in a case-management approach will be observation through completing tasks with individual clients to understand their current methods and possibly discuss alternative approaches, when relevant. For example, accompanying a client to pay a particular bill can be used for a much broader activity analysis into hygiene, appearance, social skills, use of public transport, budgeting skills and general awareness and personal safety.

ADL as a barometer of mental health

The development of a strong one-to-one relationship between a client and a case manager may occasionally enable both sides of the relationship to be more aware of the early warning signs of increased mental distress. For some people, the early signs are often decreased attention to aspects of personal care and immediate surroundings, increased isolation resulting from withdrawal from social contacts and an increasing self-neglect.

If we are considering such factors as a barometer of internal feelings of distress, we must be clear that we are observing definite changes and not simply using basic lack of skills as a meaningful indicator. This latter point must also be evaluated alongside a variety of other factors which may influence a decrease in attention to specific activities of daily living – financial problems can often result in sudden changes of priority, people on very low incomes having little or no leeway to meet the sudden requirements of a large bill or the threat of court action for non-payment. So a person may suddenly cut down on eating in order to cover the threat of the electricity being disconnected.

Motivational factors may also result in sudden changes of attention to activities of daily living. For example, a person may be making extra effort to attend to personal appearance while they are attempting to find new employment, but suddenly see less reason to maintain that standard as the chances of gaining employment look increasingly bleak or as the rejection letters build up.

COMMUNITY RESOURCES

Support services

These are offered, in different forms, by health, local authority and voluntary sector agencies. Occupational therapy assumes a prominent role, with staff located in health authority and in social service departments. The focus of functional assessment, addressing physical abilities, confidence, motivation, attitudes, social and communication skills, and the need for aids and adaptations, makes the profession ideally placed for addressing the co-ordination that is needed, particularly when resources for activities of daily living may be provided by both the health authority and the local authority.

Further health authority resources are deployed through community nursing; CPNs (community psychiatric nurse) and district nurses may offer support for aspects of personal care beyond the primary health care needs, physiotherapy, chiropody and other specialist services may also be needed to support aspects of ADL.

The primary focus of support from the local authority is through the home help organizers who make the initial assessment of home-care needs and deploying home-help and meals-on-wheels services where required. The home-help service covers a wide range of care needs – collecting pensions, shopping, cleaning and laundry – but home help organizers may be required to work with service managers to determine priorities for service provision if resources are scarce. The other potential resource through the local council is a clearance and cleaning service that may be provided by a 'dirty squad' in cases of extreme need – as was the case for Mary in Case Study 1 before she was able to return home from a hospital admission. The council may also provide a central laundry service for identified, needy local residents, accessible through the home-help service.

The voluntary sector is able to provide a wide range of services associated with activities of daily living, but they tend to be locally set up along specific lines rather than the blanket national provision of services required through statutory authorities. Examples of voluntary services range from care-attendant schemes, where people can offer help to a person at home day or night with personal care needs; volunteer accompaniment on shopping trips for people who do not have the confidence of physical abilities necessary to complete their own shopping needs; the assessment functions of a short-stay flat; to voluntary and social service day-care units which offer help and support with meals and washing machine or bathing facilities.

The role of the case manager ranges from discussion, assessment and role modelling with the client to acting as a referrer to and reviewer of other required services. They may also be able to undertake some degree of activity analysis, depending on their professional and personal skills.

The local community

By far the largest and most significant source of support for personal care and social needs is the unsung army of informal carers – relatives, friends, neighbours and the people providing day-to-day services for the local community. In addition to the individuals who may live with or near the individual clients, cafés and shops often provide an important source of contact and offers of bargains and regular meals for those on low incomes and experiencing difficulty cooking their own meals on a regular basis. These services can occasionally also offer the informal role of 'keeping an eye' on a person's general welfare, through regular contacts and conversations and alerting other local services if problems arise.

Local 'community centres' may also be invaluable for providing services of social contact, educational opportunities and the warmth and comfort of a tea or coffee bar with light snacks. Further offers of voluntary help may be provided through these centres, meeting both the needs of the client and other local people wishing to provide a voluntary service.

Other sources of local opportunities have already been mentioned in Chapter 6 – particularly help with budgeting through jumble sales, second hand purchases and charity shops.

SKILLS TRAINING OR PRACTICAL HELP?

The formal setting offered by in-patient occupational therapy departments and day hospitals have tended to focus on a problems-orientated approach to activities of daily living. The characteristics of this approach centre on referral for a problems-based assessment which will be addressed by a programme of treatment to meet specific identified needs. Drouet (1986) and McDougall (1992) outline examples of this programme development, for practical skills training and nutrition education respectively.

Frequently, a programme will centre on raising the individual's awareness, practice of skills and group discussions by using explanation, modelling, role-play, reinforcement, feedback and homework methods. Whilst such an approach is in keeping with simulated environments and the ethos of group treatment found in many of these services, it is very difficult to follow a similar approach with the individual in the community. A case manager may consider and discuss the programme for individual clients to practise skill training. However, it is often far more difficult to convince the clients of the value of their own home as a base for skills training, particularly when they are more concerned with focusing on the idea of practical help with specific tasks. Much of the practical help does take the form of training, particularly in the sense of modelling skills to the client. However, this latter point is often more easily acknowledged by the trained worker than the clients themselves.

Indeed, the strengths model of case management referred to in earlier chapters acknowledges both the limitations of a problems-orientated approach and a more specific resistance by clients to engaging in direct goal-setting to raise the standard of self-care skill (Rapp, 1988). This approach advocates the setting of goals related to the clients' strengths, but identifies the potential for improving self-care as an important secondary aim which promotes the achievement of the primary desires. For example, to focus on the appearance and hygiene factor raised in the personal profile of Bill could result in resistance because of the discomfort raised by very negative comments. However, by concentrating on the potential for achieving his desire to use the local cinema again, Bill may arrive at the conclusion himself to improve his appearance and hygiene in order to gain access to the cinema, or at least he may be reminded in a more general (and less personal sense) that people are often debarred from places of public attendance for reasons of inappropriate presentation.

In their own homes and their own communities, it is more common for a person to ask for practical help rather than demonstrate a specific need for skills training. Examples may include the following, all of which can require specific practical involvement of a case manager:

- self-care – advice on free or cheap clothing and footwear, or access to help with personal care and cleaning of clothing and bedding;
- home management – advice on cheap and second-hand furniture, home-help support and help with collecting money or budgeting;
- shopping – the support of a volunteer to accompany them, home deliveries or the option of meals-on-wheels to reduce the need for bulk shopping;
- cooking – advice on skills and safety, cheap nutritious meals and acceptance of the desire to eat out rather than cook all meals at home;
- social – the value of case-manager visits as a social function, advice on befriending schemes or community centres and drop-ins.

An important responsibility for the case manager would be that of developing an intimate knowledge of resources and opportunities throughout the local community. Occupational therapists concerned to maintain their interest in activities of daily living as a professional core function may also wish to start with McDougall (1992) as an introduction to some of the current research into the area.

SUMMARY

The term 'activities of daily living' is a wide-ranging concept. Reid (1984) suggests the need to differentiate between the basic self-care skills (physical self-maintenance) and the complex skills of social and cultural interactions (instrumental self-maintenance). Essentially the range covers the most basic motivations for personal care management, care of the home environment and the complexity of interactions with people on a social, business or emotional level.

Some of the difficulties which arise through activities of daily living may be as much a consequence of poor opportunities as they are of poor levels of skill. The case manager may need to be more attuned to the local opportunities for support than to the need for the accessibility of opportunities for skills training (Rapp, 1988; Rapp and Kisthardt, 1991).

Though the day hospital has been seen as a focal point for rehabilitative practice in the community, there is not sufficient evidence that the skills training offered there has a significant impact on community functioning. It has been suggested that a more flexible approach to individual needs be adopted in the community (McDougall, 1992), particularly through discussing the clients' own wishes, thus empowering people to assume greater responsibility for determining the types of support they may receive.

8

Day care and occupation

The title of this chapter covers a range of activities from employment to education and training, to day care services and the use of leisure. But even this categorization is too simple as each activity could be subdivided into many further parts. They are closely linked together because they share a common characteristic – each represents a different facet of purposeful activity which in turn is assumed to be a common aim shared by most people for making some use of their waking hours.

Heginbotham (1984) suggests that the linking of day care and employment is a relatively recent trend, viewing those activities as a continuum of services rather than separate entities in themselves. Thus an individual is able to achieve greater personal autonomy by moving between different activities to meet different needs, or simply finding a type of activity that feels most comfortable from personal choice rather than by professionally assessed placement.

The relationship of the elements in the chapter title is not meant to reflect any priority of service provision for this client group, nor do I wish to create an early impression that day care should be considered above and before employment for people experiencing long-term mental health problems. In line with the general philosophy of this text, we should consider individuals' wishes and abilities and realistically support them to achieve their own goals. We should look to utilize the widest range of possible opportunities, thus reflecting the real diversity of personal wants and desires.

Any assumptions held about the inability or lack of motivation of people experiencing long-term severe mental distress towards holding employment, other than sheltered employment, is merely an expression of the widely held stigma surrounding such conditions. Much of the apparent lack of motivation exhibited by individuals in this client group tends to be disinterest in the directions that other people are trying to impose. The apparent lack of motivation displayed by the person who stays in bed much of the day may possibly be a result of bed being being a more favourable option than the alternatives currently being offered.

Everybody will display degrees of motivation towards ideas and activities which hold some interest for them or more closely correspond to their personal aims. To deny an individual in this client group access to potential employment opportunities, on the grounds of experiencing mental distress and/or high unemployment in the economy, is to deny access to a basic human desire. This is particularly the case in a society which puts so much emphasis on the definition of a person by employment status.

In reality, it is difficult for many people to gain employment in times of high unemployment, but we should not be in the business of blocking all hope from the beginning, and we should not ignore the individual abilities which may just fit one of the few local openings. We should still consider a role for supporting people to learn the difficulties for themselves. If the desires are set too high we can help people to find their own realistic niche, by trial and error if necessary.

If a person realistically assesses his or her own level to be that of using day-care services and/or leisure activities with no ambitions for employment, this should be respected and supported. If people desire to engage in no purposeful activity, this position should also be acknowledged and supported if they can reasonably demonstrate that prolonged inactivity will offer less stress, where their track record of managing personally stressful levels of activity resulted in relapses of their condition.

The key is once again that of the client and helper relationship, enabling a clear understanding of the client's own aims and abilities and an openness to support expressed wishes in the context of an exploration of the potential consequences of different options for activity or inactivity.

Within this chapter I wish to examine a range of options that could be available in each broad category of activity. But, firstly, I will use a profile and case studies to illustrate some of the different standpoints adopted by individuals towards the use of their time, purposeful or otherwise.

PERSONAL PROFILE

Buki is a 49-year-old lady of Nigerian origin. Her parents and many siblings all still live in Nigeria but she has had no contact with her family for some years. Buki was married in 1965 and migrated to England with her husband the following year. They separated in 1974 when her husband returned to live in Nigeria, but he requested another man should live with her and look after her in his absence. This surrogate husband physically abused Buki on occasions until he became hospitalized (reasons unknown) in 1979.

In 1977 her two young sons were taken into local authority care having been discovered to be suffering from global language handicap, possibly resulting from social and emotional deprivation. In 1985 Buki requested that her 6-year-old daughter be taken into care because she was unable to cope with the demands of child care during periods of severe mental distress.

Buki's psychiatric history commenced in 1968 and she has experienced 11 hospital admissions in 24 years. The diagnoses have ranged from hysterical stupor to atypical affective disorder to catatonic schizophrenia. The most frequent (though not exclusive) picture is one of admission in a catatonic stupor – mute and motionless. Over variable periods of time she has gradually responded to questions, subsequently initiating more active personal care before claiming to feel sufficiently recovered to go home again. She has apparently rarely been assessed as experiencing any first rank symptoms of schizophrenia and generally initiates very little spontaneous conversation even when apparently well. The other frequent characteristic associated with most of her admissions is a physical abnormality – low blood sodium levels, generally treated by fluid intake restrictions.

Buki explains most of her admissions as a result of feeling progressively more and more tired and stressed by daily routines of activity, resulting in a need to stop all but the most basic human functions and completely resting until she feels her energy levels returning. She also attributes the periods of tiredness to a persistent experience of 'cold blood', which may probably be linked to a chronic condition of her blood metabolism. In essence, Buki describes an occasional need for temporary hibernation to regenerate her energy levels. However, these suggestions do not explain some of the less frequent episodes of bizarre, somewhat manic, behaviours in her past history.

In terms of purposeful activity Buki has an intermittent work history, begining with clerical positions in Nigeria and continuing with clerical work on her arrival in England. She has since performed a variety of cleaning jobs in offices and a local hospital and light industrial work on the production line of a canning factory. Since her last period of employment was interrupted by hospital admission in 1988, activity has focused more on day-care service options, using a local day hospital and drop-in centre.

Buki has varied her use of day care to match her perceptions of her own stress and tiredness levels – she maintains a regular weekly visit to a drop-in centre for social purposes and will occasionally join structured activities offered by the centre. She attempts to maintain attendances but will fluctuate her levels of social interaction in correlation with her perceived energy levels. Attendance at the day hospital is much more variable because of the greater demands to conform to a structured programme of activity. However, she does feel that her ability to manage the stress of the day hospital is a better measure of her ability to meet a long-term goal of returning to part-time work.

Since her daughter was taken into foster care in 1985, Buki has lived alone through a progression of council flat – women's homeless hostel – bed and breakfast hotel – temporary assessment flat – council flat. Much of this circle has been necessitated by an accidental fire in her original flat, also occasioning broken wrists as a result of jumping from the flat to escape the fire. She now feels more settled with the return of a longer-term tenancy and structures much of her time through quite rigid domestic and rest routines.

Positive characteristics

- She expresses her own personal choice of activity and routine in a more settled type of accommodation.
- She is very clear about how she uses the support of external agencies, including requesting occasional short breaks without any agency contacts.
- She is capable of using negotiating skills when she wishes to express her wants and needs, including discussing early warning signs of relapse and potential emergency plans to help offset the need for future hospital admissions.

Buki's own statement of needs:

- to engage in supervised contact with her daughter, in the hope that she may one day be able to return to live with her again;
- to remain out of hospital on a long-term basis;
- to return to part-time work;
- to maintain a consistent council tenancy that she can feel is her own home.

CASE STUDY 1

Adapting previous skills to new opportunities

Josie is a 42-year-old woman, married with three children – a teenaged boy and girl and a 7-year-old girl. She has a 15 year history of depressive illnesses with occasional suicide attempts. She has experienced five short hospital admissions with more prolonged periods of day-hospital support.

Her previous employment history commenced with six years working as a primary school teacher. Much of the last 10 years has been occupied by intermittent contact with the second-hand and antique buying and selling trade, particularly in street markets. The intermittent nature of this activity has fluctuated in line with her experiences of distress, but one unfortunate consequence has been her gradual use of the family home as storage space for items bought but not sold.

Josie was able to make some use of an occupational therapy work assessment and preparation programme, but her indecision about choosing from her available options at the end of this course led her to opt for an ongoing, but intermittent, series of supportive occupational counselling sessions. Ultimately, she was able to develop confidence in calling on her former teaching skills and took up a part-time post teaching English as a second language through a local adult education organization. She continued, with an option of visiting an occupational therapist for suppor-tive counselling, to explore her responses to the demands of the work and to reassure her own confidence in her deci-sions and abilities.

Josie quickly developed the confidence to be appro-priately critical of the organization and management of the adult education scheme (privately run). She was acutely aware of the employers' exploitation of her mental health problems through low pay, and of the poor support and supervision offered in the work place. She remained reluc-tant to seek any supportive advocacy work and remained highly critical of her own work performance, frequently expressing the possibility that she may just give it up as a bad idea.

CASE STUDY 2

Using training schemes to establish some roots

Michael is a 31-year-old single man, born in England. He has been diagnosed as suffering with schizophrenia since the age of 19, and two of his six siblings have a similar history. Frequent admissions to hospital and an unsettled pattern of accommodation changes have interrupted any attempts to establish a work record.

For Michael employment opportunities have tended to be only a few hours to a few days at a time in low-paid catering or labouring jobs. The longest period in any one activity has been three months on an introductory course to basic computer skills and a few months intermittent attendance at a local authority day centre.

One of Michael's longer-term interests has been in creative writing, inspired by his need to explain what he perceives to be previous supernatural experiences, but he does not wish to join structured creative writing groups because he feels his powerful experiences may be too frightening for other group members.

Informal discussions did open up the notion of using a word processor for documenting his thoughts and poetry. This led on to approaching a local training agency to once again consider keyboard and computer skills. For Michael, the structure of a time-limited training scheme still repesented difficulties, but the agency were able to offer informal access to computer equipment to develop keyboarding skills and computer interest outside of the formal training scheme – a kind of 'computer drop-in' was being offered to formal trainees outside the course hours and was opened up as an introductory offer for Michael.

CASE STUDY 3

When all options have been tried inactivity can still be a realistic option

Bill is a 56-year-old man, born in England and profiled in more detail in Chapter 7. Following the loss of a leg, having been wounded in action during his National Service, he became severely distressed and initially felt there would be no option for purposeful activity left open to him.

Initially, he gained a number of employment opportunities as a result of the employment quota scheme introduced in the 1944 Employment Act to ensure opportunities for disabled servicemen. He worked for periods of a few years in a briefcase assembly factory and as a lift attendant in a large office building.

As his experience of mental distress grew more severe, he found opportunities for employment more difficult to gain and felt less able to manage the pressures of structure and timekeeping. During this period of time (his late 30s and early 40s) Bill was referred to, and briefly attended, a day hospital and two separate day centres. Whilst he is able to recall gaining some enjoyment from carpentry and artwork, he generally felt little enthusiasm or interest for the structure or majority of activities and gradually became more reclusive.

Hospital admissions continued frequently and Bill became progressively more withdrawn, whichever environment he was in. For more than 10 years he has had only limited contact with the world outside his flat. He actively rejects any suggestions that entail active involvement, but will maintain contact in his own home with a limited number of people with specific supportive purposes, namely a CPN, home help case manager. He will, on rare occasions, engage in visits to places that interest him with his case manager, the most recent being a river boat trip, but he will dictate the level of involvement in activity by temporarily refusing to answer the door at times when he wishes to communicate the need for reducing or changing the level of support.

In recent years the frequency of hospital admissions has been reducing for Bill, which may be partly explained by the current range of support being pitched at an appropriate level for his needs. Purposeful activity is certainly not an item on his agenda, so the priorities for support can be currently shifted to other expressions of need.

EMPLOYMENT AS OCCUPATION

For the purposes of this chapter, these terms are not to be seen as interchangeable. Occupation is a much broader concept relating to any use of purposeful activity to structure time, including engagement in day-care activities addressed separately later. Employment is used more narrowly to refer specifically to work activity, but may include sheltered or voluntary work. So employment may be seen as just one facet of occupation.

Nothwithstanding the case of Bill, outlined above, most writers tend to focus on the dangers of inactivity for people experiencing long-term mental health problems. The work of Wing and Brown (1970) is frequently quoted. They highlighted the conclusion that inactivity in chronic schizophrenics seemed to be directly responsible for a proportion of subsequent clinical symptoms, particularly flatness of affect, poverty of speech and social withdrawal. Whilst it is difficult to argue with such conclusions, and Bill certainly demonstrates such symptoms, the question that should be addressed, in individual cases, is whether the client is truly more comfortable with this situation than the alternative stresses perceived to be inherent in structured activity and social contact. Complete solitary confinement can be avoided through appropriate levels of community support without the need to conform to higher social standards of involvement and communication.

When proposing the value of occupation in general, or employment specifically, we need to be aware of the overall context. Are we addressing the needs of the individual or the wider felt needs of society? The individual may occasionally tolerate circumstances that society in general would declare abhorrent.

The instrinsic values of work and the perceptions of why people will want to take up paid employment are widely discussed in the literature. Lloyd (1986) outlines a detailed list of the personal and physical needs that may be fulfilled by work activities, under the main headings of personal satisfaction, psychological rewards of structure and status and the inevitable financial rewards. She also suggests that it is a valuable measure of successful integration back into the local community. Acceptance by society is one of the factors also highlighted by Wansborough (1981), who suggests that stigma is reduced if you are seen as part of the homogenous, working, well population. The value of meaningful activity for promoting greater self-identity and esteem is given equal value to financial reward as a means of escaping poverty (Gilman, 1987).

Birch (1983) focuses on the wider context of the value of occupation for broadening mental activity through the need to be more social and outward looking. She suggests the alternative is 'to be idle, to have time on your hands ... time to look inwards, to worry, to look at yourself and wonder if you are ill. It is a time when small difficulties become magnified'.

Whereas much of the literature encourages us to look to the value of supporting people back into work, we must not deny that the reality of unemployment in the general workforce makes the opportunity for disadvantaged people to return to work even more difficult. Goldberg (1985) reminds us of the sense of failure that can be communicated between therapist and patient where work rehabilitation fails to produce the ultimate goal of paid employment. He suggests that we need to look into developing meaningful alternatives that can promote many of the values listed above. (These suggestions will be addressed later in this chapter.)

Birch (1983) reminds us that the successful entry into paid employment also carries intrinsic stresses and pressures: anxiety over work performances; pressures imposed through structure and time; coping with the multiple roles of worker, partner, parent; socializing and competition in the workplace; criticisms from workmates and employers; and the continuing fear of losing a job through further illness.

Despite the apparent stresses involved in participating in work-related activities, US studies into the employment of women following periods of hospitalization, reported in Bachrach and Nadelson (1988), concluded that: 'even though there was a relationship between diagnosis, treatment history and the likelihood of employment, the relationship was not strong enough to exclude psychotic individuals or those with more than five admissions from consideration'. They suggested that 'diagnosis may have more implications for the quality and type of work performance than it does for employment per se'. Gilman (1987) suggests that the role of work for structuring time and providing social contact could be considered as even more important for people suffering from long-term difficulties who find it difficult to initiate these aims through their own use of time.

So, far from being excluded from the potential work-related activity, the individuals in this client group are more likely to have their own desires met and to meet some of the professionals' treatment goals by using work as a form of treatment or rehabilitation.

For the clients (and staff) concerned about the intrinsic pressures of a return to work, it would appear as valuable to consider the support needed to keep a job as it would be to consider the support needed to find a job (Bachrach and Nadelson, 1988). Good liaison between employers and community support services can have the dual advantage of enabling the employer to seek further understanding and advice on how to cope with some of the problems encountered through mental distress, and of giving the client more confidence to approach the employer or an outside agency in times of difficulty (Birch, 1983). The case of Josie, outlined above, indicates some of the maintenance value of ongoing supportive occupational counselling. Further outreach work could possibly persuade some employers to have a more open attitude to altering employee tasks, giving some 'rest' time or holding jobs open in times of employee distress.

OCCUPATIONAL ASSESSMENT AND REHABILITATION

Assessment and rehabilitation for a return to work has been at the centre of psychiatric rehabilitation principles since the beginning of the emphasis on community care, and still remains so to this day. However, the economic recession of the early 1980s and the continued levels of relatively high unemployment into the 1990s have led to a frequent challenging of the reality of these functions (Goldberg, 1985; Heginbotham, 1985b).

There has been a resulting shift away from the predominantly hospital-based industrial workshops of the 1950s and 1960s to a broader-based community emphasis looking at all the options available. These assessments and rehabilitative practices have had to embrace the changing patterns and organization of job opportunities away from the light and heavy industry towards the expanding service industries.

As fewer and fewer rehabilitees are being placed in open employment positions, there is an increasing need to prepare people for lower paid or unpaid activities and for making purposeful use of early retirement, and to advocate for a change in society's attitudes towards the long-term use of leisure and general education in the place of work.

For the individuals in the client group who express the need to return to work as their prime objective, support is needed through the process of addressing vital questions: At what stage am I fit to return to work? What type of work am I best suited to? Who will discuss my fears and anxieties about returning to employment? (Birch, 1983; Norris, 1989). A process of supportive occupational counselling is clearly needed, to be linked to the functions of occupational assessment and rehabilitation.

Work assessment

Vostanis (1990) refers to this as 'the first stage in vocational rehabilitation. It should not only evaluate the occupational skills of the patient but it should also take into account other factors such as self care, mental state, motivation and social relationships, which are essential for a competent work performance.'

The use of an occupational questionnaire prior to the functional assessment should attempt to measure an individual's commitment to work (Norris, 1989). Combined with the results of assessment, such a questionnaire may help to guide the subsequent direction of rehabilitation initiatives.

A thorough work assessment should ideally seek to include mobility, work capacity, technical skills, communication skills, personality and intellectual capacity; it should further address financial requirements, transport difficulties and any potential workplace accessibility problems. The assessment will need to further discover if the individual has a job to return to and, if so, does it need any adapting or rewriting of job description; will the person need to retrain and, if so, how long will the rehabilitation period be likely to take; and is the individual open to considering alternative occupational options (BAOT, 1990).

The work assessment may also include the use of established psychological tests, such as the Measurement of Performance of Psychiatric Patients, the Standardized Assessment of the Work Behaviour of Psychiatric Patients and the Job Rating Scale. Full assessments may be offered through a number of health service, central government or voluntary sector skills assessment centres.

Occupational rehabilitation

In some cases, ongoing rehabilitation/training may be offered in the same location as the work assessment. For example, Worklink at Lambeth Accord offers a full three week assessment, followed by work training in specific areas such as office skills and catering. The training period may range from 6 months up to 12 months and includes more general job preparation skills and temporary placements with local employers.

Worklink shares common characteristics with other assessment and training centres (Asset in east London, Skillnet in London Docklands) in that it offers a service to local people and to a mixed range of disabilities that would include access for people with long term mental health problems. It fosters links with the local job market, matching skills with available opportunities, thus ensuring a higher rate of success for placing people into open employment as an end product. A number of health service and voluntary sector 'model' services are described by Pilling (1988) to illustrate the diversity of opportunities that could be offered to people in this client group.

In general terms, Wansborough (1981) suggests that work rehabilitation should be managed through graded steps:

- manipulate the environment according to the individual requirements of the patient;
- introduce a greater balance between patient and environment;
- the patient is able to accommodate, to an acceptable degree, to the demands of society.

To a large extent, the graded approach is the model followed by the staff of many occupational therapy units in creating simulated work environments within their departments, particularly in the use of office equipment, carpentry workshops and horticulture (though the range and diversity can vary according to staff skills and available equipment).

In addition to the practice of specific job skills, I have already referred to the inclusion of job preparation skills offered at Worklink. It is acknowledged by many that the process of finding work can be as great a challenge as the development of the skills necessary for a particular job. Work preparation skills are now widely offered as part of the rehabilitation package presented in occupational therapy departments as well as the specialized assessment and training centres. Examples of the content of these pre-work skills courses can be found in Norris (1989) and the Employment Issues Programme outlined below which attempt to help people address a range of occupational options open to them.

The Employment Issue Programme is designed to provide opportunities to explore the processes involved in job-finding and to explore the range of occupational options available. Practical experience will be offered to help develop job-finding skills and to evaluate communication skills required in the process. The objectives are:

- to investigate sources of available jobs:
  – job centres (job clubs/Disablement Resettlement Officer); notice boards; newspaper advertisements; calling; friends; temporary work agencies;
- to examine the information provided in job adverts:
  – title; pay and conditions; time; prospects and training;
- to examine the requirements for completing application forms;
- to evaluate knowledge and practice performance in interview technique:
  – preparation; techniques; barriers and stresses;
- to examine past work record with emphasis on evaluating personal work habits:
  – evaluate work skills/work habits; reasons for leaving; pressures and stresses of employment;
- to examine a range of occupational opportunities:
  – return to existing job
  – search for new employment/DRO
  – self-employment
  – further training
  – voluntary work
  – organize leisure time;
- to examine methods for structuring leisure time;
- to evaluate employers' attitudes towards the incidence of mental illness.

The programme will primarily consist of discussion groups for information exchange; verbal and non-verbal communication exercises to develop practical skills; and the use of published materials (information leaflets/application forms) for accurate and realistic content.

The programme can run over 8 to 12 weeks (depending on demand for practical exercises). The group meets once a week for a period of 1½ hours and additional individual/small group sessions can be arranged for practical sessions, such as video role-play interviews. The maximum number of patients/clients for the group is ten.

To be refered to the programme, patients/clients express a desire to gain a form of occupational status and displaying problem areas in retaining gainful employment.

OCCUPATIONAL OPTIONS

The full range of occupational options would include day care, education and the productive use of leisure and recreation (which will be discussed later), but at this stage I propose to consider many of the employment and training options that could be available. The following is not an exhaustive list but does cover many of the more frequently covered pathways, in addition to the voluntary sector assessment and training mentioned previously.

When a person has concluded that they are ready to return to a form of work, the next decisions involve a consideration of whether they wish to return to full- or part-time paid employment, a form of 'sheltered' employment, or take up the less stressful option of voluntary work. Do they wish to use existing acquired work skills, to retrain and develop new skills required by the changing job market on their own initiative, or do they wish to seek out potential support from case managers or specialist employment agency workers. Each of these decisions may have been addressd through the help of a job preparation course.

The most direct route will be to visit the vacancy boards in the local Job Centre and to study the work vacancies in the local newspapers. The Job centre is the favourable option for accessibility to the widest range of employment and training opportunities, either through a restart interview with a member of the Job Centre personnel or through an interview with the Disablement Resettlement Officer. The latter is a specific post in each Job Centre, set up under the Disablement Advisory Service and responsible to the Job Centre Manager for placing people with disabilities into jobs or training schemes. This is the post that will consider the options of registering as disabled and implementing the 1944 Employment Act quota system (Birch, 1983; Norris, 1989).

The 'Restart' interview is designed to introduce unemployed people to the range of opportunities offered through a job centre.

- Restart courses, for up to two weeks, give training in job-finding skills.
- Job Clubs, for up to two weeks, help long-term unemployed people to search for jobs by offering coaching sessions, newspapers, telephones, writing and postage materials. There is an expectation that each person will apply for a minimum number of vacancies each day.
- Short-term government training schemes.
- Self-employment through an Enterprise Allowance scheme.
- Job start allowance payments to local employers considering employing a person on a temporary assessment basis before making a decision on offering permanent employment.
- Access to local community and voluntary work schemes.
- The payment of 'therapeutic earnings' on top of normal receipt of invalidity benefit if a work opportunity is seen as an essential part of psychiatric rehabilitation.

Some of the above options are considered to be too demanding for people experiencing long-term severe mental distress because they involve open competition in the market with all other unemployed people. For this reason, historically, a number of more supported initial steps have grown and developed.

Sheltered employment

These are closely linked to hospital industrial therapy units, the industrial therapy organisation (ITO) and Remploy (Wansborough, 1981). Traditionally, these units have operated by providing sheltered industrial work and light subcontract work. Low pay is linked to continued receipt of benefits but they have gradually found less success in moving people on to open employment.

Employment rehabilitation centres

These are a government initiative organized along similar lines to the voluntary assessment and training centres discussed previously. They attempt to offer short-term placements, to reacquaint people with general work skills through practising different skills. They have tended to suffer the same difficulties as sheltered schemes, particularly through offering a limited range of opportunities, largely industrial, at a time when the skills base and work opportunities have been undergoing a change towards service industries in open employment generally.

Sheltered individual placement schemes

This was a joint initiative in the 1980s to address the problems of sheltered schemes failing to prepare for open employment. Under this arrangement, an individual is able to be placed in open employment but under sheltered conditions. A local authority or voluntary body acts as a sponsor, so the employer pays a lower pro rata rate of pay with the sponsor making up the difference through a claim via the government employment and training agency. This scheme enables people to take up placements suited to their individual needs and skills (Gilman, 1987).

User-led initiatives

User-led initiatives have tended to follow two methods so far:

1. In the US the temporary work placement scheme has been pioneered through the development of Fountain House in New York, whereby individuals are placed in open employment for up to six months then another user takes over the placement. This is a further option for offering realistic work experience before the individual decides to compete in the open job market. Fountain House also offers work experience through performing the many practical and administrative functions for its own day-to-day operations – clerical, maintenance, media and catering (Chamberlin, 1988; Pilling, 1988).

2. Co-operative employment projects have been occasionally user-led initatives and occasionally voluntary organization led. Their particular benefit has been to give a closer approximation to the changing needs of current employment trends by offering service-based functions such as painting and decorating, furniture restoration, café and sandwich bar facilities and printing services.

Voluntary work

Voluntary work is an option developed through a number of sources – government schemes, hospital projects, voluntary organization projects, user organizations. It is generally considered to be a low-stress option for structuring time productively and gaining work experience, thus enabling individuals to negotiate their own time and input to varying degrees.

Whilst the traditional concerns of industrial therapy and sheltered employment have attempted to broaden their base by branching out from light industrial and sub-contract work to packaging, assembly, engineering, craft and horticultural skills, they have still only managed very limited success in helping clients to achieve their personal goals of open employment. But there has been a gradual development of many creative training, work experience and employment opportunities growing out of government, statutory sector, voluntary sector and user-led initatives. Lloyd and Guerra (1988) have suggested that 'through the establishment of comprehensive, vocational rehabilitation programmes, the occupational therapist plays an important role in assisting the individual to prepare for work'. Whilst such a programme would include assessment, training and occupational counselling, the occupational therapist and case manager need to be aware of the wide range of occupational options locally available in order to fulfil a useful role in directing and referring clients on to other services that will help to meet their needs for work.

DAY-CARE SERVICES

This term refers to the largely formal organization of daytime care and support offered to people outside of the in-patient treatment services of the psychiatric units. Added to this would be a smaller collection of *ad hoc* informal facilities developed by the voluntary sector and service users, with or without financial and manpower resource backing from the statutory sector services.

In relation to the specific client group, day care is often seen as the priority option for providing support and rehabilitation, particularly for the people deemed by professionals and employers alike to be unemployable. This view may also be held by clients themselves who have decided they are not yet, or may never be, ready to return to employment.

Day hospitals and day centres

Historically, day care was initiated in the UK and North America through the establishment of the first day hospitals in 1946. By the 1960s a day hospital 'movement' was being acknowledged (Farndale, 1961). It remained entirely a function provided by the health service until the introduction of local authority social services departments in 1971 and the subsequent introduction of the day centre.

The DHSS (1975) White Paper, *Better Services for the Mentally Ill*, drew up a clear distinction between the different forms of day care to be offered. The day hospitals were to offer treatment-orientated facilities for short-term care under health authority control, and the day centres should give long-term social support under local authority control. Though the White Paper did acknowledge the inevitability of some overlap of functions, subsequent investigations have revealed a nationally uneven development of services. Considerable overlaps have been found to occur in function, client group and lengths of stay, and the staff development of aims and objectives (Ekdawi, 1981; Vaughan, 1985).

Despite this lack of clarity between the day hospital and the day centre, there is still quite a degree of consensus about the overall aims of day care: to provide an alternative to hospital admission, a transitional support between hospital and community, and a mix of short-term intensive rehabilitation or longer-term support depending on individual needs (Holloway, 1988; Pilling, 1991).

Vaughan and Prechner (1986) suggest that the *ad hoc* development of day care services has resulted in three separate distinguishable approaches to service delivery:

- the laissez-faire drop-in approach;
- contractual, sessional attendances;
- the therapeutic community system.

Although the different approaches clearly give rise to different staff interaction, very little research has been undertaken to measure the relative outcomes for individuals in the more disabled client group. Vaughan and Prechner (1986) report that a small study of patients with shorter-term acute episodes of mental illness preferred the contractual approach to working on specific aspects of their condition, with feelings of directionless quoted in relation to the social format of the drop-in. It is only inferred from this study that the drop-in may be more suited to the needs of the more socially isolated individuals of a more disabled group.

Other brief studies have attempted to determine what users see as the benefit of attending day units – Garvey (1991) was unable to conclude any factors with statistical significance between attenders and non-attenders, but it did point to the role of the keyworker, the quality of initial information given and whether the client perceived the service to be of value as important areas to be considered. Birch (1983) reported that many users saw day care as an alternative to work, a chance to meet others in the same position as themselves, a break from the monotony of home and the opportunity of occasionally being involved in interesting activity. She also discovered that some clients did not attend day care units because they perceived the activities to be silly and childish and the type of structure held no signifiant interest. Some of these conclusions are supported by Pilling's (1991) report of recent studies, which indicates a contradiction between the client viewing day care as an essentially social function and the staff often tending to view it as a therapeutic function.

Whatever the outcome of research activity, the fact remains that day care services meet the needs of some clients but not of others. This reinforces the requirement to be sensitive to individual need rather than being prescriptive of activity on a client-group level. Furthermore, knowledge of a wider range of services may enable a more accurate tailoring of placement to individual need.

Drop-in centres

This type of facility has grown in many different formats for varying life-spans in recent years. The professional view, that this type of facility more directly caters to the 'social' needs of the client group, has resulted in its more frequent growth in the voluntary sector and through user initiatives. However, as the statutory sector workers have increasingly recognized its value, so part of the day hospital or day centre space and programme has been given over to a drop-in function (Pilling, 1991).

Chamberlin (1988) gives a detailed description of a user-led initative developed by the Mental Patients Association in the United States. This example grew into a 16-hours-a-day, 7-days-a-week facility, with temporary paid co-ordinators from amongst the users, and a democratic structure of management through every user having an open invitation to weekly business meetings.

Hope and Pullin (1985) describe how the Oxford Mental Health Association developed 'The Mill'. From a lowly beginning centred on the kettle and ashtray, users were gradually encouraged to develop their own interests and abilities to use the centre in many different ways, as they wished. This has been an example of a voluntary sector initiative developing through the collaboration of users, volunteers and interested professionals. 'The Mill' is reported to have achieved its primary goal of providing a place of interest for users to visit. The secondary goals of developing individual abilities and activity tends to fluctuate.

A Mental Health Users' Centre, initially established within the grounds of Hackney Hospital before subsequently moving out to suitable community accommodation, is an example of a statutory service initiative, operated through staffing by community service volunteers. Supervision of the volunteers through the occupational therapy staff, and management through a multi-disciplinary committee guided its development. The users clearly responded to the low degree of structure offered by a drop-in service and to the volunteer staff. The initiative was principally set up to target a large number of people who frequently returned to the hospital out-patient department, even when they did not have an appointment, presumably as a source of social contact and to escape the monotonous isolation of staying at home. Many of these clients had been identified as finding some difficulties accepting offers of more structured day-care services. The aim became one of re-engaging people at the initial place of their choice – near to the hospital out-patient department and using volunteers who would not be as closely identified with the roles of professionals – then gradually attempting to transfer whatever functions and activities materialized back out to a community site.

The 10.00 a.m. to 4.00 p.m., 5-days-a-week facility very soon became well used, with a focus around the kettle, ashtray, music, informal conversation, games and newspapers. It should be noted that the main source of difficulty and complaints came from other hospital staff based close to the centre, particularly regarding noise and the potential abuse of drugs and alcohol on the hospital site.

Out of hours services

One of the expected results from an internal evaluation of the Hackney drop-in facility was user expression of the need for social support during the evenings and weekends – times of the week traditionally ignored by the statutory day-care services. It is generally left to the voluntary sector to cover what are often referred to by staff as the 'anti-social' hours.

A number of individual projects have grown to tackle this problem at a local level. In the case of Hackney, a long-standing arrangement has been the Psychiatric Rehabilitation Association 'restaurant club' (Wing and Morris, 1981). This has been an attempt to address the dual problems of social isolation and the provision of a cheap and nutritious meal. The club is open from 5.30 p.m. to 9.30 p.m. each evening, providing a very cheap meal in a 'restaurant' atmosphere. Adjoining the restaurant is the shared facility of a PRA (Psychiatric Rehabilitation Association) day centre, with television and social and physical fitness activities available. Users are expected to pay an annual club membership fee as well as the cost of the individual meals.

Other evening or weekend facilities generally tend to follow the basic drop-in style of informal social contact but are frequently dependant on the goodwill of volunteers and staff to give up their time, which inevitably leaves them in a constant state of uncertainty.

Focus, clarity and co-ordination

Pilling (1991) suggests that one of the advantages of the drop-in over the formal day unit is its clarity of purpose. Any development of specific functions tends to grow out of user requirements, from very basic beginnings and with a strong degree of flexibility to meet changing expressions of need.

Conversely, the formal day unit is often subjected to internal and/or external pressures to meet multiple needs, treatment and social, for a wide range of clients. The early description of the Kirkdale Resource Centre in Sydenham, South London (Bumstead, 1985) reflects a desire to meet all needs: the day needs of the 'new long-term adult mentally ill'; short-term therapy for emotional and situational disturbances; a mental health information centre; an advisory resource; a source of support for families and friends of the client; an educational centre for professionals working in mental health; and a drop-in facility for a few people who find structure difficult to manage.

Kirkdale has grown in to a valuable resource for its local area, but the danger of a lack of focus and clarity of purpose is a frequent failure to meet the needs of the more disabled client group, particularly as staff are attracted to the apparently fashionable options of verbal therapies in a way that often excludes the long-term group from participation. Poor focus at the planning stage inevitably leaves the facility to develop according to staff needs rather than client needs.

The recent development, in the UK, of community mental health centres is a similar reflection of the need to meet a diverse range of needs with the remit of a single unit. The aims and objectives set out to meet a range of local day-care needs, with specific assessment and therapy functions, an office base and/or meeting place for other voluntary organizations and, in some rare instances, the provision of a few beds with 24-hour crisis nursing care (Holloway, 1988). A current criticism is that, once again, the needs of the most disabled will potentially be lost in the attempt to address the wider needs of the local community.

Planning and co-ordination are equally as important over the geographical area to ensure that specialization in separate units is still planned to meet the priorities of different client groups. There is an equal danger that staff in separate units may decide on similar professional interests, thus excluding large areas of service need.

LEISURE AND EDUCATION

These two areas of activity are addressed together here because they may be linked on occasions, such as when leisure pursuits intrinsically improve an individual's education. It is also acknowledged that the two can be mutually exclusive, as when the activity of education is being purposefully addressed in pursuit of work.

Most definitions of leisure link it specifically as a complementary function to employment – time available free from the obligations of work; activities which may be used for rest, amusement, expending energy, improving education, being creative or socializing (Willson, 1984). It is seen as time free from the impositions of external agencies, free from remuneration, to be used for pleasure, for relaxation and/or stimulation.

I am more concerned with the question of whether leisure and education can be used as a substitute for work, to fulfil many of the aims of work perceived by the client group and society in general. Despite the frequent protestations that people in this client group should have equal opportunity of access to work, further reservations are expressed that at times of generally high unemployment those people with the additional disadvantage of long-term mental distress cannot realistically expect to compete for a finite number of jobs. Eloquent statements are made about the need to usher in a new attitude towards remuneration for other forms of meaningful activity, particularly liberalizing attitudes towards the use of leisure and education as a long-term replacement for work without the heavy financial penalties entailed in survival on social security benefits (Heginbotham, 1985b; Goldberg, 1985).

Conversely, there is a feeling that even with a liberalizing of attitudes a person is still unlikely to achieve the same degree of acquired status, productive self-image or complete community integration without some form of work (Lloyd, 1986). It is also regarded as unlikely that leisure alone could provide sufficient amounts of activity to be able to structure the day for any lengthy period of time (Pilling, 1988).

Many individuals in this client group have found themselves currently excluded from a great variety of leisure pursuits, partly through the symptomatic difficulties experienced – poor concentration and difficulty in socializing – and also because of the financial costs of the activities themselves, the need for transport, the lack of locally available resources or the unintentional exclusion of individuals if not accompanied by partners or if they are not part of the established teams.

Without major shifts in society's attitudes, access to resources and removal of the financial disadvantages, leisure will continue to be seen as an adjunct to other forms of work or day care for occupying and structuring time. Access to sports centres and community centres, to libraries and special interest groups can help to rekindle interest in activity and give a focus to the use of some spare time, but rarely can they be anticipated to structure anything in excess of 35 hours a week. Encouraging creative activities, such as a wide range of writing or playing musical interests, will similarly organize relatively small amounts of time, except for the few who are able to pursue an interest across the boundary of leisure into the realm of work, when very significant amounts of time are required to be devoted to the practice of any activity.

In the case of adult education services, efforts have been made to minimize the costs for more disadvantaged people. Whilst a wide range of practical and academic interests are promoted, very few people would seriously see this as an option for providing the main structure to their time as a replacement for work. Access to Open University study may come closer to meeting this requirement but, again, the client will need to be supported through the careful consideration of the pressures involved in taking on such a commitment.

THE FUNCTION OF THE CASE MANAGER

As with most other areas of client wants and needs covered in this text, the case manager has a number of supportive roles to offer to the individual – counsellor, adviser, companion and advocate. In addition to the one-to-one contact, a great deal of writing, telephoning and meeting will be required on a day-to-day basis.

There will be a need to develop a wide range of knowledge of opportunities available in the local area, to act as a personal resource for clients. In addition to discussing specific interests, people in this client group may often benefit from a worker accompanying them on the initial visits to new facilities until the person feels sufficiently settled and confident to attend alone.

The role of advocate may extend beyond representing the specific needs of an individual to advising the relevant authorities of identified gaps in current services. In exceptional circumstances, the case manager may be considered to have the skills and the expert knowledge of the client group needs to fill a gap in day-care services, for example, development of a low-key drop-in facility or different forms of more formal support groups. The skills of the occupational therapist would equip them to fulfil such a role, though it would not be a role exclusive to one profession. However, the decision to take up such function needs to be evaluated against the reduction in time to meet other service requirements.

SUMMARY

Purposeful activity is universally proposed as a vital form of support for people who have experienced long-term severe mental distress (Willson, 1987). The range of options for purposeful activity covers a wide variety of day care and occupation (Birch, 1983). However, the option of relative inactivity should not be summarily dismissed until we fully appreciate the desires and needs of the individual.

Despite the undeniable advantages conferred by the structure, status and financial rewards of employment (Lloyd, 1986; Gilman, 1987), it is not a realistic option for many disadvantaged people in an age of relatively high unemployment

(Goldberg, 1985). More credence needs to be given to the occasional call for a radical review of our attitudes towards offering greater financial incentives to those that focus more on day care, leisure, education or even socially useful activities such as voluntary support and environmental conservation (Heginbotham, 1985b; Goldberg, 1985).

Community support through day-care services should be flexible in its approach to individual needs and co-ordinated on an area-wide basis to ensure different requirements are able to be addressed and scarce resources are not squandered through duplication. More professional staff should acknowledge the value of the drop-in facility, both for its intrinsic functions and as a way of developing more formal services as an evolving response to genuine user needs (Pilling, 1991).

Case managers have a number of roles they can offer in respect of day care and occupation, but they can also lead the development of a positive outlook towards the local community as a source of support, rather than narrowing the focus of activity into stigmatized mental-health only services (Rapp, 1988; Rapp and Kisthardt, 1991).

9

Advocacy and user empowerment

The focus of the previous chapters of this book has been on the practical approaches that 'workers' can pursue to meet the needs of service users, hopefully, with the emphasis usually on the needs expressed by the clients themselves, through assessment or consultation processes. It is now vital to conclude with a review of the developments that are of primary importance in the priorities of users and user groups – how best to articulate individual and collective user needs and how to ensure that the provision of services accurately reflects the identified needs. Within the scope of this chapter I also propose to review the debate surrounding the role of the professional regarding advocacy issues and user-led initiatives.

'Advocacy' and 'user empowerment' are terms that have been in use in the mental health field throughout the 1980s in the UK but date back to the early 1970s in the USA – a brief historical overview is presented below. For some non-users (carers, workers, managers) these terms are merely considered to be current buzz-words, but the 'flavour of the month' has been around for far too many months to be simply dismissed as a passing fad or fashion. For others, they have become the most significant developments in mental health services, as reflected by Barker and Peck (1987) with their suggestion that 'people who have been devalued and disempowered can only start to be restored to full citizenship if the power imbalance between users and providers is redressed'.

Historical developments in the 'User Movement'

North America
Late 1940s   WANA (We Are Not Alone) – later to develop into Fountain House, New York.
1970   Insane Liberation Front, in Portland (Oregon).
1971   Mental Liberation Project, in New York.
              Mental Patients Liberation Front, in Boston.
              Mental Patients Association, in Vancouver (Canada).
1972   Network Against Psychiatric Assault, in San Francisco.
              Madness Network News – began as a San Francisco area newsletter but grew into a national network newsletter.
1973   Conference on Human Rights and Psychiatric Oppression – held annually until 1985; users and ex-users only from 1976.
Late 1980s   Two distinct national organizations coexist:
              (i) National Alliance of Mental Patients – opposition to all forms of forced treatment, and (ii) National Mental Health Consumers Association – more conciliatory stance towards the mental health system.

United Kingdom
1975   Promotion of Rights of Mental Patients
1980   COPE – user run counselling service in West London.
              Campaign Against Psychiatric Oppression.
1982   British Network of Alternatives to Psychiatry.
1985   World Mental Health Congress, in Brighton.
1986   Survivors Speak Out.
              Conference of users in Nottingham and Newcastle invite Dutch advocates to speak of their experiences.
              Patients Councils develop in Nottingham.
              MIND National Conference more open to users of services.
1987   National Advocacy Network Conference.
1988   MIND Consumer Network, with the MINDLINK newsletter.

The need for advocacy and user empowerment is highlighted by Chamberlin (1988) when she suggests that 'our ideas about ''care'' and ''treatment'' at the hands of psychiatry, about the nature of ''mental illness'', and about new and better ways to deal with (and truly to help) people undergoing an emotional crisis differ drastically from those of mental health professionals'. It is becoming widely recognized that users should be increasingly valued more as individuals in their own right. This includes being able to determine their own labels in preference to the stigma-loaded labels of the psychiatric professions, such as chronic, psychotic, schizophrenic. The 'user movement' is becoming increasingly regarded as a force with which professional service providers should openly participate in order to support the growth of radical new services which genuinely meet user needs.

Not all people share the optimism of this latter point. There are significant numbers of workers who hold somewhat irrational fears which can only be likened to the persecutor's fear of being persecuted and which blocks any attempts to negotiate a partnership. Some of the fears would appear to be founded on the misplaced notion that, given the opportunity to speak, users can speak of nothing but the negative ideas of radical anti-psychiatry. Linked to this is the more widespread fear of losing power as a result of the need to share and compromise. The concept of power will be discussed shortly, and it is understandably at the centre of the notion of user empowerment.

Before we address the above issues in more detail, I would like to discuss briefly why this chapter should be included in a book largely devoted to 'practical approaches'. You may be forgiven for thinking the subject matter belongs more to the realms of conceptual thinking rather than practical achievement, but closer inspection reveals the contrary: the aims of much of 'therapy' are to promote the independent articulation of the clients' needs and to develop the practical skills in order to function more independently in meeting and satisfying these needs. In this light, the ideas of self-advocacy and user empowerment, outlined in this chapter, represent the epitome of expressing needs and seeking practical means to achieve those needs through the involvement of the user.

Furthermore, this chapter is central to the whole concept of this book, because much of the development of the concepts of advocacy and user empowerment has been through specific practical projects, not rhetoric, to meet real needs rather than perceived needs. A part of this chapter will subsequently focus on the 'complementary' and 'alternative' practical solutions to those traditionally offered by professional services.

POWER

In general terms, the idea of power relates to having the ability to carry out actions or to instruct others. In the context of mental health services, it relates to the ability to exercise choices regarding the fundamental aspects of one's own life: to be in control of the decisions which will directly impinge on the individual, from the most basic day-to-day needs (what to eat, when to eat, when to sleep) to the more complex long-term decisions (where to live, how to occupy the time, what relationships to encourage).

Thus, we can begin to see that the power does not just relate to positions of authority such as Prime Minister, Chief Executive of a business corporation or Principal of a college. Whatever occupational position you hold, why not take a few moments now and consider the power you can exert – what choices and what decisions are you personally in control of, particularly regarding your own life?

Disempowered users feel they have no control over, or choice about, how they live, relate, or manage their own experience of distress. The psychiatric system has historically adopted a suppressive approach wherever personal choice is concerned. Even meal times, bed times, the need for communal sleeping arrangements have been dictated, generally, in the name of the more efficient management of the psychiatric unit. So efficiency in terms of staff needs has all too often subsumed personal choice and dignity in terms of patient needs. Chamberlin (1988) gives a graphic portrayal of being disempowered by the mental health system in the USA in 1966. Many users in Britain and America would argue that little has changed over the ensuing 25 years.

The overall result of this disempowerment is to create a feeling of being thoroughly devalued as an individual. This comes in addition to the underlying distress that may have brought the person to the attention of the psychiatric services.

The mechanism on which power in mental health services is based is 'information', the tool with which to make informed choices. But in order to be of any use, information needs to be freely accessible, complete and presented in an understandable way. This latter point is very important because it would be easy to make just token gestures by purporting to give information, but in a deliberately obscure manner that renders it unintelligible to the service user. So our own use of language, particularly jargon, needs to be addressed when we aim to present information to service users with the intention of supporting informed choices. Most professionals will recognize the need to be 'bilingual' – well versed in professional jargon – to create the impression of being a 'member of the club', but will recognize also the need to occasionally explain our work in plain language. In reality, only the latter is necessary.

Freely accessible information can often be very difficult to obtain, partly because the holders fear a partial loss of power. The 'consumer movement' already has a long history of struggle to gain access to information, often having to resort to litigation in order to bring about the release of necessary information. Nader (1973) gives a good account of the tasks facing the consumer movement in the face of corporate power.

In Britain, even with the advent of the Data Protection Act 1985, the Access to Personal Files Act 1987 and the Access to Health Records Act 1990, there is still much debate over access to confidential information. There also seems to be great variation between different organizations about how open their information is to service users. This in turn necessitates more administration because of the need to seek permission in many cases, before information can be exchanged. I do not wish to continue into this minefield any further at this point, but I would advise any student on placement or new worker to familiarize themselves with the local issues of confidentiality and information exchange.

The day that we achieve greater uniformity of rules across information systems cannot come too soon. In the meantime, we need to work with the fears that are held around the sharing of information. We must also guard against the danger of information sharing becoming too one-sided, where users are expected to divulge all their thoughts, fears and needs, whilst workers continue to claim privilege of access to their own analysis of data. Barker and Peck (1987) point to 'one of the bi-products of this process of users taking responsibility and thus speaking for themselves is that the resulting information can be used for service evaluation purposes', but immediately highlight this as 'the process of empowerment and not an end in itself'. We must be open to freely sharing the results of evaluation as well as the knowledge picked up from professional education that can benefit the service users' attempts to achieve dignity and independence.

At this point, it is important to note that restricted access to information and feelings of disempowerment in mental health services are not exclusive to service users. Many workers can find themselves disempowered through a lack of information filtering down the hierarchical structure. It is a rare occurrence, but not unheard of, for a user of a particular service to be more aware of the plans for that service than the workers, through membership of a Community Health Council or other lobbying body. Let us not lose sight of the fact that any example of worker disempowerment would have to be greatly magnified before they begin to express the feelings encountered in user disempowerment.

AUTHORITY

Power is a central theme to the discussions in this chapter but, in many cases, alongside the possession of power through holding information must go the ability to exercise that power. Permission to use power can be delegated through the concept of 'authority'. This is most easily understood by considering the hierarchical structures of large organizations, whereby any number of personnel may have access to 'classified' or privileged information, but only some may have the authority to use or communicate the information. This is particularly seen in the case of those who, within the organization, may communicate with the local or national press.

Let us not see this solely as a facet of large organizations; it is an all too common characteristic of any organization or groupings of people that there will be some implicit authority to use the power vested in the group by certain individuals – the natural leaders will always have a habit of emerging.

WHAT IS ADVOCACY?

In general terms, the process of advocacy has grown out of the legal system of representation, where a legal professional will represent the views of a client within the legal process.

The momentum for introducing advocacy into the area of mental health service provision is not entirely related to mental health law. Rather it is because the system has, in many ways, failed to meet the expressed needs of those it seeks to serve. More specifically, Meteyard (1990) suggests

'advocacy is necessary because inevitably:

- errors arise from judgements made by resource controllers;
- all services not given as a right are open to interpretations and these can be disputed;
- some services are very expensive and/or scarce;
- national and local policy or statutes may be vague and open to misinterpretation.'

A general definition of the process of advocacy might be 'the communicating of expressed needs by, or on behalf of, a client to the service providers'. But within this concept there are widely differing types of advocacy.

Self-advocacy

Defined by MIND (1990) as 'a process in which an individual, or group of people, speak or act on their own behalf in pursuit of their needs and interests'. It requires people to value themselves and to take positive action to challenge their devalued status in the eyes of the psychiatric system and wider society.

Citizen advocacy

Defined by MIND (1990) as a method of enabling 'disadvantaged people to be paired with ordinary citizens who will support them in obtaining their basic human rights'. It is seen as a service to be provided to people who are unable to safeguard their own rights, where the advocate represents the other person's views as if they were his or her own. Primarily a citizen should help the person to achieve self-advocacy, where possible.

Legal advocacy

The provision of professional legal representation, either in relation to the complex matters of Mental Health Law or to help overcome the barriers and delays that psychiatric diagnoses can present to the normal access to legal services for criminal, family, property, employment, immigration or consumer law. Only legal advocacy is a paid service, though legal aid schemes are available to support access to the system for people suffering financial hardship.

Some of the citizen advocacy projects have started life sponsored by statutory service initiatives, but subsequently broken away to become independent. As Renshaw (1987) explains, this latter development is essential to the growth of the citizen advocacy movement in order to provide the basis for objective comment on the services provided to clients. Sometimes the statutory services have responded to citizen advocates in a critical manner (Robson 1987), seeing them as 'troublemakers' and challenging their claim to be objectively representing a client over and above their own personal opinions. In Holland, the integrity of its citizen advocates is ensured by employing them all through a 'National Foundation of Patient Advocates'.

Despite having the efficacy of their role questioned by professionals and some user groups, most citizen advocates tend to agree with the assumption that the desired goal should be that of promoting the achievement of self-advocacy for all users of mental health services. Much of the discussion in this chapter focuses on the achievement of self-advocacy groups, but I will also later explore some of the debate which surrounds the question of whether professionals can genuinely claim to any type of advocacy role.

Advocacy and user empowerment are two very distinct, but mutually bound, entities. Advocacy, as seen above, can be interpreted in a clearly defined way as the communication of the needs of service users to service providers and planners. User empowerment, on the other hand, is a much broader concept which requires a much more fundamental change of attitudes and behaviour from service users and services providers.

USER EMPOWERMENT

This is a relatively self-explanatory term which describes a process of giving more 'power' to the users of the service in the form of information and the ability to express choice. But, if we are to do it any justice, we must acknowledge from the outset that this is a very complex, wide-ranging subject which can have a number of different interpretations. In its simplest form, it would require professionals to ask individuals their needs and views. It also encompasses many shades of information giving and sharing, leading to the establishing of mechanisms which promote full and active participation in service planning, provision and evaluation.

User empowerment has grown from an understanding of 'consumerism' and the earlier growth of the consumer movement in response to the power of the commercial and industrial organizations. The need for such a process in the area of mental health is the result of a wide 'power differential', most clearly expressed by the traditional views of the 'active worker' and 'passive patient' roles. In this scenario the professional is believed to know what is best for the service user and exercises all the choice over what will be received.

Barker and Peck (1987) discusses how workers can carry some long-established prejudices, including a lack of confidence in the ability of users to think and act responsibly for themselves. Both training and work experience narrows their focus of attention to seeing the user as a set of problems to be treated. Thus, user empowerment as a process requires significant changes of attitudes before a practical change in behaviour can be expected. This attitude change can begin with a fresh approach to training, but Barker and Peck (1987) also indicate that attitudes can be changed through experience, demanding a greater openess to new ideas and partnership with service users.

Growing, as it does, out of a tradition of suppressing user views, the process of empowerment will also require a significant change of attitudes on behalf of users, particularly people who have experienced long-term difficulties and contact with services. They have not been traditionally used to being seriously asked what they want or need, so expectations of being listened to would have to be radically altered. Hutchinson, Linton and Lucas (1990) suggest that 'involving users in planning mental health services is an acknowledgement that they have a rich wealth of knowledge that can be used to guide, inform and advise ... professionals and users should meet on a more equal basis ... where users are not permanently cast in the sick role'.

The most significant barrier to implementing the ideas engendered in user empowerment is the workers' fear that they will lose some of their existing power. This fear appears to be based on vague assumptions that power is a commodity in finite supply which requires those currently with the most power, to relinquish some to those with the least. Differing opinions are understandably voiced on this issue: Renshaw (1987) suggests that putting these ideas into practice will require hard thinking and the overcoming of challenges, and also that for 'professionals it means giving up some of their power – not an easy move or gesture to be made lightly'. On the other hand, Beeforth *et al.* (1990) suggest there is evidence to indicate that successful partnerships between user groups and service providers can actually result in an overall increase of power.

Whichever viewpoint is held on the resulting redistribution of power, there is still a need to consider the appealing argument by Beeforth *et al.* (1990) that co-operation needs to be given a chance in order to compete for scarce resources and to meet the competitive tendering for service contracts that will characterize the new 'market' influence in the provision of health services.

There are no consensus views held on advocacy, user empowerment or consumerism between user groups, let alone between users and workers. But Barker and Peck (1987) suggest that as long as user interests are not subsumed under worker interests, the conflicts can have positive outcomes through a new clarity of thinking – where workers can respond more sensitively to user needs and users feel they have a stronger power base from which to declare their views.

Another major pitfall to guard against when considering the process of user empowerment is the possibility, conscious or otherwise, of producing only token gestures in practice. There may exist a general appeal for workers and managers to talk about consulting the user – useful statements to include in planning documents and operational policies. There may even be very real discussions held where users are asked their opinions. But if we find that behind the bold statements of intent there are no clearly stated actions for carrying the results into practice, it is likely to amount to negative results of anger and frustration. Hutchinson, Linton and Lucas (1990) suggest that to conform to the prevailing climate without real commitment is dishonest, and destructive to users who may have believed their contribution was genuinely welcomed.

It is important that professionals are quite clear as to how they intend to implement consultations and the subsequent changes to practice. Hutchinson, Linton and Lucas (1990) suggest that most people intend to undertake user involvement correctly, but it should not be rushed into lightly. They also warn against over concern to get everything exactly right – this may just be a delaying tactic resulting in yet another token gesture. The important thing is to get the process started and not to delay it on the basis that we don't know precisely how to proceed.

THE QUESTION OF PROFESSIONAL INVOLVEMENT

The complexities of the issues are again raised when we consider what roles the professionals may play with regard to advocacy and user empowerment. Not only are there wide-ranging points of view on the subject, but we must once again separate out two very distinct questions which are nevertheless closely interrelated, namely:

- What advocacy services can professional workers offer to their client groups, if any?
- What form does the user and worker partnership take in order to promote greater user empowerment?

Advocacy and the mental health professional

If there is to be any advocacy role for mental health professionals it would not fit easily into the models outlined earlier, those of self-, citizen and legal advocacy. The first prerequisite is that of independence in order to represent the views expressed by the user clearly to the service providers.

In the most common case, that of representation to the mental health service themselves, it is obvious that the professional will find it impossible to achieve an independent standpoint for the following reasons:

- The employment contract and job description legally obligate the worker to the functions specified by the employer.
- The organization's budgetary constraints may impose specific guidelines on the working methods and priorities to be followed by its employees.
- Much of the education, training and work experience of the professional will hinder his or her ability to adopt and represent the users views without some degree of argument or modification based in a personal perspective and assessment.

There is still, however, the question of the ability of the mental health professional to independently represent needs in areas outside specific issues of mental health but impinging directly on the experience of distress, namely housing and personal finances. The likelihood is that these areas will also be influenced by training, i.e. the necessity to make a professional assessment of need which may differ markedly from the perception of the user. We should also be open to the probability that an individual user will reveal different pieces of information to those they perceive to be wholly independent than they would to a professional – and each set of information may form different parts to the whole jigsaw.

Some writers do hint at the possibility of advocacy roles to be fulfilled by professional workers; Meteyard (1990), in looking at specific roles that a keyworker could play, suggests three examples where they may intervene in the system on behalf of the service user:

- where disputes arise between service user and and agency;
- where services are rationed and there is competition between users for scarce resources;
- where circumstances change or worsen.

He also suggests that even where these advocacy roles are established, the professional worker still needs to be aware of falling into the critical traps of over-representing one or two individuals or user groups, at the risk of being criticized for not offering such services more widely.

These comments suggest that there is a limited advocacy role to be played, despite the issues over independence. But, we should not lose sight of the notion that the ideal situation is the promotion of self-advocacy groups. Advocacy should certainly not be seen as the new high-profile role that professionals can try to usurp from service users. Ideally, professionals should stay within the parameters of their own expertise but should be encouraged to be more open and responsive to the growing voice of self-advocacy. They can have a limited active role but should leave the specialist functions to those best suited to the task, i.e. primarily the users themselves.

Before we leave this subject, it is necessary to consider also the specific client group to whom this book is addressed – those people who find difficulty in vocalizing their own needs and gaining access to services representing their needs. Again the mental health professional has a duty to continually lobby for more resources to meet the demands of this disadvantaged group. Rather than assume a specialist advocacy role on the misguided assumption that user representatives neglect the more disabled individuals, professionals would be better placed to be the link to enable access to self-advocacy services.

User empowerment through partnership

As we have seen earlier, the concept of user empowerment requires changes in attitude and behaviours from both users and workers. Where conflicts tend to arise is over what form the ensuing collaboration should take.

Chamberlin (1988) outlines three models that have been followed in attempts to provide alternative services:

- The partnership model – professionals and non-professionals collaborate, but the traditional distinction is upheld between those who give and those who receive help.
- The supportive model – non-professionals have equal rights with users but professionals are only permitted external roles, e.g. writing letters of support.
- The separatist model – all professionals and non-professionals are excluded, so users and ex-users of mental health services provide support exclusively for each other.

The 'case for separation' is fully explained by Chamberlin (1987); she argues that it grew in the 1970s in the USA out of dissatisfaction with all the efforts made by workers to collaborate with, and empower, service users. But she also hints that British experience shows some potential for the unique strength of the convergence of survivors and radical workers.

Other more wide-ranging views have been expressed on the potential for partnership. In the supportive model, Chamberlin (1988) sees the possibility of professionals providing a figurehead role to ensure credibility in the eyes of funding agencies and bureaucracies.

Beeforth *et al.* (1990) suggest that professionals be encouraged to work within the existing structure of their organizations to lobby for greater support and understanding by their managers and service planners so that greater user involvement may take place throughout the structure of the service.

In some cases, there is now full collaboration where professionals are invited to user-group meetings to share information and knowledge and to lend manpower support for administration tasks, such as minute-taking and distributing publicity information. In these cases, it is generally conducted with the expressed understanding that the professionals have no voting rights. It is vitally important, from the onset, that the roles and relationships be clearly defined between the users and the workers and, even in these circumstances, users should still hold regular meetings where all non-users are excluded. Chamberlin (1988) suggests the rationale of holding separate meetings is that the important function of consciousness-raising is not possible if non-users are present because of their innate attitudes towards mental distress, however well-intentioned they may be as individuals.

What becomes clear is that no ideal model exists for collaborating to promote user empowerment, and local circumstances and personalities will influence the adoption of different solutions. On a positive outlook, Beeforth *et al.* (1990) suggest that 'empowerment does necessitate risks for all ... the risks may be far outweighed by the enriching experience of users and paid working collaboratively and sharing experiences ... one possible outcome is, as reported by both professionals and users, a launch into some of the most creative and interesting work ever undertaken'.

CASE STUDY 1

Advocating outside the mental health services

Mehmet is a 32-year-old man of Turkish Cypriot origin who has lived in the UK for approximately 20 years. He has been in frequent contact with the mental health services since the age of 17, but the most alarming situation has been during the last three years, including serving a one year stay of an 18-month sentence in prison following a conviction for actual bodily harm and a number of short stays in a locked psychiatric unit.

Mehmet's priority need on release from prison was for suitable accommodation. He found that he had un-expectedly lost his tenancy of a one-bedroom flat. Just to intensify the situation, after an alleged incident in a temporary bed and breakfast placement, the council housing department suspended their responsibility for housing this man (Section 72 (b) of the Housing Act 1985) on the grounds that he was a convicted arsonist with a history of fire-raising.

The pertinent facts here are that two separate fires had taken place in council flats in Mehmet's tenancy. He explains the first as an accidental use of candles after his electricity had been cut off (he was rehoused by the council after this incident), and no charges were made against him. The second fire apparently occurred whilst he was detained in prison. Mehmet had also used threatening behaviour to the staff of a 'Homeless Persons Unit' and assaulted members of the public; he was not charged on either occasion.

As a mental health professional offering community support, I was asked by Mehmet to help re-establish a council tenancy. It became necessary to adopt an advocacy role in two ways: to accompany other health service staff in discussions with the 'Homeless Persons Unit' in order to plead the case for a stable home base for Mehmet to help him to re-establish his own life and make use of the community support offered; to find a competent legal advocate specializing in housing and mental health issues and to support Mehmet's factual discussions in order to consider the possibility of legally challenging the assumptions on which the housing department's decisions were based.

Mehmet's only options during these protracted proceedings was to use direct access homeless persons hostels and to sleep rough.

You will be correct in assuming that there are many other details about Mehmet's needs and circumstances not discussed here. The point of this presentation is to show that it is quite possible for a mental health professional to adopt advocacy roles in issues outside of their employing agency and their direct area or responsibility. There were other options open to Mehmet for employing an advocate: he was particularly aware of the Citizen's Advice Bureau as an option, though not of any local self-advocacy groups. He chose to ask the health authority staff with whom he had been in regular contact since his release from prison. As a health professional, I found no particular conflicts in taking up such a role, though there was a degree of pressure from the housing department that the health authority should take responsibility for ensuring the stability of any future tenancy that may be established.

CASE STUDY 2
A dilemma presented by an advocacy role within the mental health services

Joseph is a 32-year-old man of Kenyan origin who has lived in the UK for approximately 10 years (his circumstances are discussed in more detail in Chapter 6). At the time of considering an advocacy role, the circumstances Joseph presented were those of recent convictions on charges of criminal damage and petty theft, with further outstanding proceedings for non-payment of court fines, non-payment of mail order debts and a charge of actual bodily harm which included jumping bail restrictions.

During a number of discussions about the frequency and increasing severity of the incidents Joseph was becoming involved in, he declined to give any explanations about the reasons for their occurrence. He also showed an erratic attendance at appointments, despite their being arranged for times and places he requested. His attention to physical health and appearance showed neglect, and though he made occasional references to being distressed he could not explain his concerns or needs with any clarity.

The one consistent request he made of my services was to explain to the necessary authorities that each of the charges resulted from periods of mental health difficulties and that he should be cleared of any charges on these grounds. My response was to suggest that he consider engaging in psychiatric treatment for a mutually agreed short term (2–3 months) to see if he was able to explain the consequences of his actions any clearer. Joseph didn't believe that I could stay with an agreement on a short-term basis, refused to acknowledge that he had any underlying mental health problems, began to disengage from any relationship with me and continued with actions that began to worry neighbours to the point of threatening retaliation against him.

My concerns were being split between helping Joseph to find the outcomes that were suitable for him and being aware of the potential threats to and by other people. I consequently felt a need to recommend that the courts consider psychiatric assessment above the option of imprisonment or further fines.

In this situation, the adoption of an advocacy role becomes blurred by perceived professional responsibilities and the influence of past experience and training. The client was requesting an advocacy role to help him achieve some important short-term goals, but the professional feels a stronger need to consider the achievement of longer-term gains, even if it results in short-term costs as perceived by the client. In these circumstances, an independent self-advocacy service is essential, and as a professional I could not honestly make a claim to an advocacy role.

PRACTICAL ACHIEVEMENTS

What follows in this section is not meant to be an exhaustive list of achievements by the user movement. It does however give an indication of what can be achieved when service users are permitted resources and the freedom to exercise choice and initiative. An important point to remember is that each of these developments represents a response to needs expressed by users themselves and not as perceived by the assessment of others. Some are entirely user-owned and led, some involve degrees of worker collaboration, a few depend on management collaboration, but all deserve our consideration and support.

Consciousness-raising

This is an essential process for the initiation and continuing development of the user movement. Consciousness-raising was adopted by mental health users following its use in promoting the growth of the women's movement. It is described by Chamberlin (1987, 1988) as a process in which 'people share and examine their own experiences to learn about the systems in which their lives are embedded'.

Consciousness-raising has probably been the single most important factor enabling users to conclude that their problems and difficulties are not exclusively internal and personal symptoms of illness but a response to real pressures and experiences in their daily lives. It is an ongoing process which enables each participating individual to renew confidence and self-esteem and challenge the stigma and stereotyping associated with mental illness. Even where there is a degree of partnership between users and professionals, it is still essential to hold regular consciousness-raising meetings that completely exclude non-users. Acceptance by professionals of the importance of this need constitutes a further step towards greater empowerment.

Support to hospital patients

Informing patients of their legal rights

People detained in hospital involuntarily should be informed of their rights, including those of appeal and access to tribunals, immediately they are admitted. As this is most likely to be a time of great distress, it is questionable how much they understand in the circumstances. User groups have attempted to provide an extra safeguard by making contact with detained patients and repeating the discussions informing them of their rights when the heat of the moment has passed.

Challenging the laws of commitment

Out of the process of consciousness-raising have come many stories of involuntary admissions to hospital where the person has felt abused and mistreated by the system. It is argued that the powers to detain people are greatly over-used because of society's stereotyped view of mental patients as being sick, unpredictable, dangerous, unable to care for themselves and unable to judge their own best interests. Such an abuse of the mental health laws is upheld by user groups as a strong reason for challenging and repealing such instruments of control. They invoke the words of Szasz (1961) who suggests that the only proper role for psychiatry in a free society is to work with individual consenting clients. Objections from the field of traditional psychiatry are countered with statements such as 'two hundred years of institutional psychiatry have shown that mental hospitals cannot help the unwilling. Incarceration is not treatment' (Chamberlin, 1988).

Visits to psychiatric units

This is a particularly important activity for informing patients of alternative forms of support available when they are discharged, for raising thought-provoking issues not adequately addressed in hospital rehabilitation and treatment programmes and for supporting the development of patient councils.

Patients councils

These are hospital ward meetings for residents only, where the patients feel free to vocalize genuine feelings about their day-to-day environment and where such views can be represented to hospital management through a hospital council made up of ward patient representatives and management representatives. Issues for discussion may range from hospital signposting and complaints about menu choices to plans for hospital closures and the replacement facilities in the community. The first development of its kind in the UK took place in Nottingham from 1985, with the first hospital council meeting in September 1986. Nottingham has further consolidated the process by developing a patient council support group, devised to help people to set up their own meetings in the psychiatric units (Gell, 1987). Members of this support group may also take the role of chairing the hospital council meetings.

Community facilities

Residential services

These include campaigning against further institutional practices in the psychiatric service and some voluntary sector housing provisions, and the provision and management of housing by users for users, run on an entirely democratic and non-profit making basis. (See Chamberlin, 1988, for a description of the Mental Patients Association residences in the USA.)

Employment co-operatives

As we have seen in Chapter 7, employment is another area fraught with the obstacles of stigma of being an ex-psychiatric patient, particularly if you have a long history of difficulties. It has been equally difficult to establish employment initiatives because of the lack of funding support. Users of services have generally had to join together in the form of small co-operatives, finding a small niche through identifying a localized need, e.g. printing services or furniture restoration.

Crisis centres

Chamberlin (1988) gives a detailed description of an 'alternative' service through her own experience of the Vancouver Emotional Emergency Center. The idea is to provide intensive emotional support to people experiencing crisis, a true form of asylum where people can deal with the pain of their distress in a personal supportive environment rather than be processed through the secure and institutional environments of the psychiatric system.

Drop-in centres

A true drop-in should not be seen strictly as an aspect of services provision but rather as a location for focusing the growth of a supportive community. It should be run on democratic grounds with equal responsibility assumed by all those wishing to be involved. Participation should be entirely voluntary, encouraging involvement by each individual only in the activities of their choice. Disputes should be resolved by the same democratic processes of negotiation and decision-making as are used in other aspects of the centre.

Community yellow pages

This is a particular project developed by Lambeth Link Self Advocacy Project in South London, whereby the most basic and useful information on community services is presented in a usable booklet for patients on discharge from the local hospitals. It provides names, addresses and telephone numbers of employment projects, advice centres for housing mental health and specific ethnic group services, social services offices and leisure and educational facilities in the local area. Additionally it provides basic advice on financial matters, and an introduction to the self-advocacy project.

Medication leaflets

Statutory services, and psychiatrists in particular, are often criticized for not giving adequate information to their patients about the ways in which medications work and the possibility of experiencing side-effects. Lambeth Link Self Advocacy Project is one example of a user's organization that attempts to redress this issue of poor information by presenting a series of leaflets outlining some of the necessary basic information, and giving access to other organizations that may be able to provide further advice and information to people worried about how prescribed medication may affect them. It should be noted that the style of presentation in these leaflets is likely to do more to encourage the taking of medication rather than promoting non-compliance.

Crisis support card

Very much in the vein of organ-donor cards, Lambeth Link Self Advocacy Project has developed a small foldaway card for use if an individual is experiencing a mental health crisis in a public place. It outlines vital information that others should take into account, such as how to contact a specific nominee/ advocate, current medication, telephone numbers of recognized user groups and any other points of importance to that individual. This should be sufficient information to aid supportive management of a crisis in the manner chosen by an individual user.

Exchanging telephone numbers

This is the simplest method for users of services to provide mutual support. It only requires the making of a personal decision about who to disclose your number to, but it has occasionally been hampered in the cases of group therapy, where professionals tend to emphasize the importance of keeping within the boundaries set by the times of group meetings.

Organization and management

Consultation and representation in planning mental health services

More frequently now, individuals and user groups are being invited to sit on committees, join planning groups and working parties. Some organizations, such as MIND, are specifically writing into their constitutions the need for user representatives on committees. Generally, these developments are made with the genuine intention of including the views of recipients in the development of the service.

Employment interview panels

A new development is the inviting of representatives of user groups to be part of the interview panels for different professionals joining mental health teams. This will make a valuable contribution to focusing the minds of prospective job applicants on the issues of user empowerment, but it will also depend in part on the powers of veto that a user representative can exercise on the decisions of a wider panel.

Self-advocacy projects

Lambeth Link has already been mentioned as an example of a local group developing projects to meet the needs of local people. There are currently approximately 150 such groups located in the UK, operating independently to develop their own projects to reflect local ideas and expertise in meeting locally identified needs.

Regional and national advocacy networks

A logical step to strengthen the identity of a 'movement' is for local groups to send representatives to meet those of other groups sharing a common purpose. Rather than follow the administrative boundaries defined by national and local government, advocacy groups are attempting to liaise in more naturally occurring regions. One such example is the newly developing South London Advocacy Network, covering user groups in each of the South London Boroughs. The groups have also now developed a national network of representatives with an annual national conference.

Bill of rights/patients charter

Irrespective of international boundaries, the development of user movements has always thrown up a common concern of basic human rights being denied to people with a history of mental health problems. A number of statements have been developed by different groups to declare an entitlement to certain rights and to promote the principles of user empowerment. One such example is Charter 90, developed by Lambeth Link in consultation with local users of services (a shortened version of Charter 90 appears in the Appendix).

Training

Conferences

This aspect of training involves invitations to speak at a wide range of conferences concerned with mental health issues.

Initiating workshops

Lambeth Link Self Advocacy Project has again been very active in promoting a series of workshops each year, reflecting the important issues and concerns in mental health. The most important feature of these workshops is an attempt to encourage equal attendance by users and non-users in order to share views and experiences. Users are beginning to be offered a more prominent role in the training of professionals, a development which must increase if professionals are to adopt a more realistic stance in response to real experiences.

These have only been examples of the work being developed by pioneering self-advocacy projects. There is still enormous scope for these ideas to be accepted and implemented more widely and, in their own modesty, the pioneers are open to seeing further improvement of the current ideas.

Again it must be stressed that it is not for the professionals to seize control of these developments but to openly encourage their wider adoption and to support the power of the users to continue to exercise choice and initiative.

The UK user movement has grown rapidly, and this momentum can be continued through appropriate professional support and, more vitally, through the adequate resourcing of self-advocacy. Beeforth *et al.* (1990) recommend independent funding from central funds, administered locally, for self- and citizen advocacy. At a time when the whole structure of health authority and local authority provisons are undergoing radical change, the opportunity should not be overlooked for giving such proposals full support, both in the financial sense and that of a commitment through the underlying values of service provision.

The 'long-term' client group

Whilst the user movement actively challenges the use of labels such as 'long-term', preferring to champion the right of individuals to determine their own labels, we must not get caught up solely in the ensuing intellectual discussions and consequently avoid the more difficult practical challenges that these people present to user advocates and workers alike. If the quality of society is measured by its responses to the most vulnerable citizens, then, likewise, the quality of a mental health system (including users, advocates, workers and managers) must be measured by its articulation and response to the needs of the most vulnerable clients.

Far from being only representative of the most articulate users, the user movement has involved and reflected a great deal of the needs of the more disadvantaged individuals. Many of the above practical achievements offer benefits for people across a wide spectrum of experiences of mental distress.

Although the growth of self-advocacy is the preferred situation for all, the option of independent citizen advocacy has its merits for initially articulating the views of some people who find it less easy to speak for themselves or join groups. Professionals still have a vital role in identifying some of these people and helping them gain access to appropriate advocacy services. For some time yet, the professionals will continue to have a limited advocacy role to play in promoting the improvements in health and welfare by these individuals.

SUMMARY

The ideas of advocacy and user empowerment are based on separate but interrelated concepts, whereby users and non-users of mental health services can be positively encouraged to express their views in the knowledge that they will be listened to and acted upon favourably. The concepts have become necessary because ideas about 'care', the nature of mental ilness and ways of supporting people in emotional distress differ markedly between the users and the professionals (Chamberlin, 1988).

The 'power' to make decisions and exercise personal choices lies at the heart of the conflict in the area of mental health (as in many others areas of human interaction). In order to distribute power more equitably, professionals will, firstly, have to overcome their own fears of apparently losing some of their power (Renshaw, 1987) and, secondly, make information more freely accessible, complete and understandable, in order that informed and meaningful choices can be made by the service user.

Barker and Peck (1987) suggest that successful user empowerment requires significant attitude changes by the professionals, through fresh approaches to their training and a greater openness to new ideas and partnerships with service users. The attitudes of service users would equally need to undergo some changes, most especially in terms of raising their expectations of being adequately informed and listened to. Hutchinson, Linton and Lucas (1990) point to a richer wealth of knowledge becoming available to the service planning mechanism if professionals and users could be encouraged to meet on a more equal basis.

The role of the professionals in providing advocacy services and promoting greater user empowerment remain quite ambiguous. Meteyard (1990) highlights a role in cases of rationing scarce resources, but the professional can never lay a claim to objective independence because of the values inherent in their training and the economic ties of employment (Chamberlain, 1988). Ideally, they should lobby for greater user involvement within the structures of their employment organizations (Beeforth *et al.*, (1990). Chamberlain (1988) also offers the suggestion of an initial figurehead role, in a supportive model of collaboration, in order to provide the unfortunate need for credibility in the eyes of funding agencies.

No ideal model exists for collaborating to promote user empowerment. Local circumstances and personalities will initially influence the development and adoption of solutions. Beeforth *et al.* (1990) point to the potentially attractive aspects of taking the inevitable risks of sharing power through meaningful collaboration. Many radical and successful ideas are implemented through the development of self-advocacy groups, and although the professionals should refrain from attempting to adopt such ideas as their own, they have a responsibility to offer a link for service users into such projects – particularly in the case of people with long-term mental health problems who may have found greater difficulty accessing such services personally.

10

Conclusions

Traditionally the people experiencing long-term mental illness have been seen as a collective of individuals defined by reference to the problems they exhibit and by the poor expectations they engender in others. First and foremost they are referred to as the chronic group, the long-term mentally ill, the unmotivated. They may often only be referred to as 'people' at a secondary level, and very rarely are referred to as people with positive attributes and abilities (Lavender and Holloway, 1988; Pilling, 1991).

A more positive focus needs to be created in workers' attitudes. Only then, will we be able to begin to successfully address some of the wants and needs, wishes and desires that are regarded as important by the very people who experience severe mental distress (Rapp and Kisthardt, 1991). This process can begin by learning to value people as individuals with their own perceptions and potential abilities, their own particular motivations and personal desires. It is not a question of ignoring problems or denying the existence of personal difficulties, but rather a more positive reframing of our skills in observations and assessment. Perhaps, more importantly, we need to develop a whole new line of questioning that enables us to examine the more positive attributes of an individual's set of experiences, and not just inquire into the occurrence of problems.

The most common factor that characterizes this diverse range of individuals is the apparent experience of complex multiple needs and unmet desires. It may be argued that service providers from a wide range of professional back-grounds have failed to meet such complex needs. However, many of these individuals have tended not to respond favourably to establishing multiple relationships with professionals from different backgrounds in order to fulfil different sets of needs (Onyett, 1992).

Holloway (1988) has suggested:

> There is a need to have at the heart of any system of care a team whose specific task is the welfare of the continuing care client. ... Care to the individual is best co-ordinated by a keyworker or case manager, who organises a package of support, using a variety of agencies. This package will be based on an individual assessment of need and a sensitive understanding of the person's inner world ... There is a clear challenge to professionals to develop a flexible, accessible and informed community support service that assertively seeks to engage those in need.

A case management response embodies all the above elements of engaging with the client, jointly assessing what is required and providing and co-ordinating a package of services to meet individual needs (Ryan, Ford and Clifford, 1991; Onyett, 1992). The personal strengths model of case management has been developed as a specific method of focusing the attention of the relationship on to the clients' wants, wishes, desires and abilities, rather than the problems and disabilities (Rapp, 1988). This model implies that a problems-orientated approach to rehabilitation potentially suffers from the trap of concentrating the client's energy on past failures which presents a negative base from which to generate motivation (Weick *et al.*, 1989).

The personal strengths approach highlights the vital importance of engagement as the first function to the helping process (Rapp and Kisthardt, 1991). If insufficient time and effort is given to the development of the working relationship, the subsequent assessment outcomes will necessarily be more limited, one-sided and intrinsically negative in outlook. Rapp and Kisthardt (1991) also highlight the significance of an outreach method of working; this is seen as a positive method of promoting client empowerment, signalling a genuine intention to work with people on their own terms and in their preferred locations.

Rapp and Wintersteen (1989) suggest the potential outcomes of the strengths model are positive changes through the successful achievement of client-agreed goals: reduced frequency of hospital admissions, reduced lengths of hospital admissions, fewer traumatic and negative contacts with services, and the meeting of needs that genuinely impact on the immediate quality of life of the individual.

The suitability of the occupational therapy profession to the personal strengths method of working arises from the value it places on the need to establish a close therapeutic relationship with the individual client (Lloyd and Maas, 1991; Brown, 1991) and the acknowledgement of using a client's strengths in order to address the difficulties that arise from the problems-orientated assessment. Craik (1991) suggests that the profession should not be held back by introspection; the progression of individuals into care management enables occupational therapy to be represented at the heart of new developments in health and social care.

The more significant current debate is whether case management should be developed by individuals undertaking postgraduate training to attain the broader range of skills necessary or whether a new profession could be developed. Kanter (1989) indicates the importance of the specific attitudes and aptitudes of individual workers, making them suitable or unsuitable for the challenges of working with this particular client group.

The evidence suggests little need to abandon existing professional curricula in favour of a new generic profession. It seems much more realistic to expect individual professionals, from whatever background, to seek out in-service training and postgraduate experience of the special interest in this client group. This can only continue to enrich the service by a continuous drawing on interest from a wider source. The role of unqualified workers and users as case managers is much less clear. These represent equally valuable resources to be considered in pursuit of the most flexible and appropriate packages of support to people in this client group.

Some of the most radical developments in community mental health are currently being offered by user groups and the greater involvement of users in the training of professionals (Chamberlin, 1988; Beeforth *et al.*, 1990).

User empowerment can only realistically grow, on an individual and a collective basis, if the professionals are prepared to undergo a shift of attitudes and share power of choice and decision-making through sharing more information. This need not involve any particular loss of role or professional credibility. Hutchinson, Linton and Lucas (1990) summarize the position as follows:

> It is very important to realise that involving users does not imply that service providers are redundant or have no skills – rather that they need to use their skills in a different way in order to empower users, themselves and their colleagues. The skills are those of working with people rather than for them; of listening and acting on knowledge gained rather than responding to people's diagnoses or 'labels'; of establishing jointly agreed individual care programmes and networks of support instead of channelling people into the current limited services.

The advocacy role that professionals could perform for service users should remain limited to improvements in housing conditions and financial circumstances. The issue of independent judgement precludes them from being able to realistically advocate on issues that would bring them into conflict with their own employers and specific job descriptions, let alone the philosophy developed through their own professional training (Chamberlin, 1987). A more vital role may be the support of self-advocacy groups by enabling members of the most disadvantaged client group to access the services of existing user-led self-advocacy schemes. Additionally, professionals could adopt a responsible attitude through supporting the need for funding the development and growth of self-advocacy groups.

Good quality community service and support should ideally arise from the creative and flexible use of local resources (Rapp, 1988; Rapp and Kisthardt, 1991). In the UK the development of community care over the last 30 years, in this and other client groups, has been considerably patchy and uncoordinated when viewed from a national perspective. Whilst still acknowledging the vital importance of the individuality of local circumstances, there have been significant calls for greater central budgets to fund the development of community care

(Kings Fund College, 1987), which could give the initiatives the national prominence they need in practice and not just in political statements.

The UK experience of the late 1980s and early 1990s has seen two major new developments transfer from the US – models of intensive case management for people with long-term mental health problems and the steady growth of the concept of user empowerment. The most important task for the remainder of the decade should be the closer linking of these two ideas, with the aim of adopting a more co-ordinated policy of community care that would be more responsive to meeting the needs and desires of individuals in this most needy client group. Although only a little progress is being made in determining the causes of persistent severe distress, we are all able to co-operate with the aim of promoting greater personal choices. Significant improvements could be made in the quality of life experienced by individual people living in the community, with the real exception of achieving more personally meaningful roles.

Appendix

EXTRACTS FROM 'CHARTER 90'
(LAMBETH LINK SELF ADVOCACY PROJECT)

1. Origin and Purpose of the Charter.

It is a statement of the rights, needs and aspirations of people experiencing mental distress, irrespective of ethnic origin. It is intended to serve as an essential source of reference for the relevant authorities in determining relations with and providing culturally sensitive services for such people.

2. Philosophy.

Mentally distressed people should have the same basic human rights, to life, and to personal security to meet their physical, mental, social, cultural and emotional needs as other people. It is crucial that no one has to accept the label 'mentally ill' in order to receive services.

3. Consultation

A range of good services for people experiencing mental distress will only be developed if distressed people are consulted and positively encouraged to express their needs in a sensitive manner.

4. Human and Civil Rights.

Personal liberty is undermined by fears of compulsory detention and treatment. If compulsion is necessary, it is essential that the person be informed of their rights and given opportunity and support to challenge the decision.

5. Information and Participation.

Services should provide realistic choices in a cultural and gender context to users about how they wish to live their own lives and should provide the information necessary to make an informed choice.

6. Care and Treatment.
i) People have a right to a personal, human approach.
ii) People have a right to a real choice of treatments.
iii) Users, their relatives and/or advocates should be given full information about medication, and other forms of treatment, including information about their possible effects, whether beneficial or harmful, in a simple clear way.
iv) The users, however severely distressed, have a right to consultation and choice about proposed treatments.
v) In view of the serious medical and social consequences of some psychiatric diagnoses, users should be given details on what the diagnoses mean and also how they can contest their diagnoses.
vi) The threat of withdrawal of services (including drug medication and other treatments) should not be used because of lack of communication due to language difficulties, nor as a form of punishment when making assessments.

7. Access to Services.
Agencies that provide services to those in mental distress should be widely publicised. Those who operate a referral system should ensure that they accept self-referrals and increase the number of agencies that can submit referrals.

8. Crisis Accommodation.
There needs to be a full range of residential alternatives to hospitalizations. These should provide safe havens that are culture and gender specific.

9. Housing.
It is essential that a full range of accommodation is offered and there is full consultation, involvement and information about what is available to users, caring relatives and/or advocates in the appropriate language.

10. Crisis Intervention.
Culture sensitive strategies must be developed to deal with the need to intervene in the lives of people actually in crisis.

11. Medical Care.

People who experience mental distress should be given the same right to medical treatments as anyone else, and not discriminated against.

12. Occupation, Employment, Education and Leisure.

i) It is vital to appreciate that all forms of occupations including leisure and sport activities can play an important part in creating well-being and fostering positive mental health.

ii) Educational and Vocational Training courses as well as social skills training should be available to people who have experienced mental distress.

iii) The council and all statutory and voluntary agencies should strive to be culturally and gender sensitive about the employment and occupational needs of people who have experienced mental distress.

iv) Practical steps should be taken to actually create opportunities for meaningful and dignified employment, both inside and outside of hospitals and day centres. Employment of patients should not be exploitative.

13. Welfare Benefits.

People who have experienced mental distress and are eligible for welfare benefits should be given practical help, support and advice in claiming the benefits they are entitled to.

14. Social Life.

Services should support the social life which the distressed person has already established rather than isolating them or breaking their existing networks of support.

15. Support for Carers.

More attention and resources need to be paid and offered to carers. Information on financial, practical and emotional support is required and should be widely advertised in different languages.

16. Access to Information.

All information about users rights and service provision must be freely available to any user, his/her relatives and/or advocates in the language that is most appropriate culturally to that user.

17. Closing of Large Hospitals.

People living in the large hospitals have the same right to self-determination, cultural and gender development and security as people living in the community. This means that, at the very least, provision has to be made to offer them a choice of a better refuge by which we mean, non-medical, humane, safe and culturally appropriate caring places where people can explore their own experiences in a protective environment, in their own time.

People in special hospitals have the right to a non-punitive, culture sensitive therapeutic environment.

The above extracts from 'Charter 90' are published with the kind permission of the Lambeth Link Self Advocacy Project.

References

Allen, T. (ed.) (1990) *Care Managers and Care Management*, Policy Studies Institute, London.

Audit Commission (1986) *Making a Reality of Community Care*, HMSO, London.

Bachrach, L.L. (1988) Defining chronic mental illness: a concept paper. *Hospital and Community Psychiatry*, **39**(4), 383–8.

Bachrach, L.L. (1989) Case management: toward a shared definition. *Hospital and Community Psychiatry*, **40**(9), 883–4.

Bachrach, L.L. and Nadelson, C. (eds) (1988) *Treating Mentally Ill Women*, American Psychiatric Press, Washington.

Barker, I. and Peck, E. (eds) (1987) *Power in Strange Places*, Good Practices in Mental Health, London.

Bayliss, E. (1987) *Housing: The Foundation of Community Care*, MIND and the National Federation of Housing Associations, London.

Bebbington, P. and Kuipers, L. (1988) Social influences on schizophrenia, in *Schizophrenia: The Major Issues*, (eds P. Bebbington and P. McGuffin), Heinemann, Oxford, pp. 201–25.

Beeforth, M., Conlan, E., Field, V., Hoser, B. and Sayce, L. (1990) *Whose service is it anyway?*, Research and Development for Psychiatry, London.

Birch, A. (1983) *What chance have we got?*, MIND, London.

Birchwood, M., Cochrane, R. and Moore, B. (1988) Family coping behaviour and the course of schizophrenia: a follow-up study. Submitted to *Psychological Medicine*.

Birley, J.L.T. and Brown, G.W. (1970) Crisis and life changes preceding the onset of relapse of acute schizophrenia:

clinical aspects. *British Journal of Psychiatry*, **116**, 327–33.

Bowden, R. (1991) Power to the user. *British Journal of Occupational Therapy*, **54**(8), 281.

Brandon, D. and Towe, N. (1989) *Free to Choose: An Introduction to Service Brokerage*. Good Impressions Publishing Ltd, London.

Brent-Smith, H. and Dean, R. (1990) *Plugging the Gaps: Providing a Service for Homeless Mentally Ill People*, Lewisham and North Southwark Health Authority, London.

British Association of Occupational Therapists. (1990) *Occupational Therapists Reference Book 1990*, Parke Sutton, London.

Brough, A. and Craig, C. (1985) Lambeth Housing Department Special Needs Section, in *Good Practices in Mental Health Housing Information Pack, Good Practices in Mental Health*, London.

Brown, M.M. (1991) *Community Mental Health Occupational Therapy: An Exploration of Distinctive Qualities*, British Association of Occupational Therapists, Unpublished Thesis.

Bumstead, C. (1985) The Kirkdale Resource Centre: a new model of community adult mental health care. *British Journal of Occupational Therapy*, **48**(10), 305–6.

Carpenter, W. and Heinrichs, D. (1983) Early intervention, time-limited, targeted pharmacotherapy of schizophrenia. *Schizophrenia Bulletin*, **9**, 553–62.

Carpenter, W., Hanlon, T.E., Heinrichs, D.W. *et al.* (1990) Continuous versus targeted medication in schizophrenic out-patients: outcome results. *American Journal of Psychiatry*, **147**(9), 1138–48.

Chamberlin, J. (1987) The case for separation: ex-patient organising in the United States, in *Power in Strange Places*, (eds I. Barker and E. Peck), Good Practices in Mental Health, London.

Chamberlin, J. (1988) *On Our Own*, MIND, London.

Clifford, P. and Craig, T (1989) *Case Management*, Research and Development for Psychiatry, London.

Craik, C. (1991) Once an occupational therapist. *British Journal of Occupational Therapy*, **54**(10), 369.

Creek, J. (ed.) (1990) *Occupational Therapy and Mental Health: Principles, Skills and Practice*, Churchill Livingstone, Edinburgh.

Creer, C. and Wing, J.K. (1988) *Schizophrenia at Home*, 2nd edn, National Schizophrenia Friendship, London.

Davis, A. (1985) Confronting poverty, in *Life After Mental Illness? Opportunities in an age of unemployment*, MIND Annual Conference 1984, MIND, London, pp. 14–16.

Day, R., Neilsen, J.A., Korten, A. *et al.* (1987) Stressful life events preceding the acute onset of schizophrenia: a cross-national study from the World Health Organisation. *Culture, Medicine and Psychiatry*, **11**, 123–205.

Department of Health (1989) *Caring for People: Community Care in the Next Decade and Beyond*, HMSO, London.

Department of Health (1991) *Implementing Community Care*, HMSO, London.

Department of Health and Social Security (1975) *Better Services for the Mentally Ill*, HMSO, London.

Drouet, V.M. (1986) Individual behavioural programme planning with long-stay schizophrenic patients. *British Journal of Occupational Therapy*, **49**(7), 227–32.

Eakin, P. (1989a) Assessments of activities of daily living: critical review. *British Journal of Occupational Therapy*, **52**(1), 11–15.

Eakin, P. (1989b) Problems with assessments of activities of daily living. *British Journal of Occupational Therapy*, **52**(2), 50–4.

Ekdawi, M.K. (1981) The role of day units in rehabilitation, in *Handbook of Psychiatric Rehabilitation Practice*, (eds J.K. Wing and B. Morris), Oxford University Press, Oxford, pp. 95–8.

Etherington, S. (1983) *Housing and Mental Health*, MIND and Circle 33 Housing Trust, London.

Falloon, I.R.H., Boyd, J.L. and McGill, C.W. (1984) *Family Care of Schizophrenia*, Guilford Press, London.

Falloon, I.R.H., Boyd, J.L., McGill, C.W. *et al.* (1985) Family management in the prevention of morbidity of schizophrenia. Clinical outcome of a two year longitudinal study. *Archives of General Psychiatry*, **42**, 887–96.

Farndale, W.A.J. (1961) *The Day Hospital Movement in Great Britain*, Pergamon Press, Oxford.

Fernando, S. (1988) *Race and Culture in Psychiatry*, Tavistock/Routledge, London.

Finlay, L. (1988) *Occupational Therapy in Psychiatry*, Croom Helm, London.

Frankland, M. (1991) The story of Freddie the Weaver, *Observer* 12 May 1991, London.

Gabell, M. and Bevan, P. (1985) Claybury/Circle 33 assessment flat, in *Good Practices in Mental Health Housing Information Pack*, GPMH, London.

Garety, P. (1988) Housing, in *Community Care in Practice: Services for the Continuing Care Client*, (eds A. Lavender and F. Holloway), Wiley, Chichester, pp. 143–60.

Garety, P.A. and Morris, I. (1984) A new unit for long-stay patients: organisation, attitude and quality of care. *Psychological Medicine*, **14**, 183–92.

Garvey, C. (1991) Factors influencing attendance and non-attendance at a day unit. *British Journal of Occupational Therapy*, **54**(7), 249–52.

Gell, C. (1987) Learning to lobby: the growth of patients' council in Nottingham, in *Power in Strange Places*, (eds I. Barker and E. Peck), Good Practices in Mental Health, London.

Gilman, S. (1987) Alternatives to open employment in the community. *British Journal of Occupational Therapy*, **50**(5), 158–60.

Goldberg, D. (1985) Rethinking rehabilitation, in *Life After Mental Illness? Opportunities in an age of unemployment*, MIND Annual Conference 1984, MIND, London, pp. 8–10.

Goldberg, D.B., Bridges, K., Cooper, W. *et al.* (1985) Douglas House: a new type of hostel for chronic psychiatric patients. *British Journal of Psychiatry*, **147**, 383–8.

Goldman, H.H. (ed.) (1988) *Review of General Psychiatry*, Prentice-Hall, London.

Goodwin, S. (1989) Community care for the mentally ill in England and Wales: myths, assumptions and reality. *Journal of Social Policy*, **18**(1), 27–52.

Griffiths, R. (1988) *Community Care: An Agenda for Action*, HMSO, London.

Harris, M. and Bergman, H.C. (1988) Misconceptions about use of case management services by the chronic mentally ill: a utilisation analysis. *Hospital and Community Psychiatry*, **39**(12), 1276–80.

Hawkins, P. and Shohet, R. (1989) *Supervision in the Helping Professions*, Oxford University Press, Buckingham.

Heginbotham, C. (1984) *Webs and Mazes*, Centre on Environment for the Handicapped, London.

Heginbotham, C. (1985a) Good practice in housing for people with long-term mental illnesses, in *Good Practices in Mental Health Housing Information Pack*, GPMH, London.

Heginbotham, C. (1985b) *Life After Mental Illness? Opportunities in an age of unemployment*, MIND Annual Conference, MIND, London.

Hirst, L. (1988) *High Care Housing*, SHIL (Single Homeless in London working party) and SITRA (Specialist Information and Training Resource Agency for single person housing), London.

Holloway, F. (1988) Day care and community support, in *Community Care in Practice: Services for the Continuing Care Client*, (eds A. Lavender and F. Holloway), Wiley, Chichester, pp. 161–86.

Hope, J. and Pullen, G.P. (1985) The Mill: a community centre for the young chronically mentally ill – an experiment in partnership. *British Journal of Occupational Therapy*, **48**(5), 142–4.

Hopson, S. (1987) The principles of the activities of daily living, in *The Practice of Occupational Therapy*, 2nd edn, (ed. A. Turner), Churchill Livingstone, Edinburgh, pp. 52–81.

House of Commons Social Services Committee (1985) *Second Report on 'Community Care with Special Reference to Adult Mentally Ill and Mentally Handicapped People'* (HC 13 1984–5), HMSO, London.

Howat, J., Bates, P., Pidgeon, J. and Shepperson, G. (1988) The development of residential accommodation in the community, in *Community Care in Practice: Services for the Continuing Care Client*, (eds A. Lavender and F. Holloway), Wiley, Chichester, pp. 275–96.

Hughes, J. (1990) *An Outline of Modern Psychiatry*, 3rd edn, Wiley, Chichester.

Hutchinson, M., Linton, G. and Lucas, J. (1990) *User Information Pack: From Policy to Practice*, MIND South East, London.

Johnson, D.A.W. (1988) Drug treatment in schizophrenia, in

Schizophrenia: The Major Issues, (eds P. Bebbington and P. McGuffin), Heinemann, Oxford, pp. 158–71.

Johnstone, L. (1989) *Users and Abusers of Psychiatry*, Routledge, London.

Joice, A. and Coia, D. (1989) A discussion on the skills of the occupational therapist working within a multidisciplinary team. *British Journal of Occupational Therapy*, 52(12), 466–8.

Kanter, J. (1988) Clinical issues in the case management relationship, in *Clinical Case Management, New Directions for Mental Health Services*, (eds M. Harris and L.L. Bachrach), Jossey-Bass, San Francisco.

Kanter, J. (1989) Clinical case management: definition, principles, components. *Hospital and Community Psychiatry*, 40(4), 361–8.

Kay, A. and Legg, C. (1986) *Discharge to the Community: a Review of Housing and Support for People Leaving Psychiatric Care*, Housing Research Group, The City University, London.

Kings Fund College. (1987) *Making a reality of Community Care: response to Sir Roy Griffiths and his review team*, Kings Fund College, London.

Lakhani, B. and Read, J. (1990) *National Welfare Benefits Handbook*, (20th edn), Child Poverty Action Group, Great Britain.

Lavender, A. and Holloway, F. (eds) (1988) *Community Care in Practice: Services for the Continuing Care Client*, Wiley, Chichester.

Leff, J.P. and Isaacs, A.D. (1990) *Psychiatric Examination in Clinical Practice*, Blackwell Scientific Publications, Oxford.

Leff, J.P. and Vaughn, C.E. (1981) The role of maintenance therapy and relatives expressed emotion in relapse of schizophrenia: a two year follow-up. *British Journal of Psychiatry*, 139, 102–4.

Leff, J.P. and Vaughn, C.E. (1985) *Expressed Emotion in Families*, The Guilford Press, New York.

Leff, J.P., Wig, N., Ghosh, A. *et al.* (1987) Influence of relatives expressed emotion on the course of schizophrenia in Chandigarh. *British Journal of Psychiatry*, 151, 166–73.

Liberman, R.P., Mueser, K.T., Wallace, C.J. *et al.* (1986) Training skills in the psychiatrically disabled: learning coping and competence. *Schizophrenia Bulletin*, 12, 631–47.

Littlewood, R. and Lipsedge, M. (1989) *Aliens and Alienists: Ethnic Minorities and Psychiatry*, 2nd edn, Unwin Hyman, London.

Lloyd, C. and Guerra, F. (1988) A vocational rehabilitation programme in forensic psychiatry. *British journal of Occupational Therapy*, **51**(4), 123–6.

Lloyd, C. and Maas, F. (1991) The therapeutic relationship. *British Journal of Occupational Therapy*, **54**(3), 111–13.

Lloyd, K. (1986) The Bec Enterprises Workscheme. *British Journal of Occupational Therapy*, **49**(8), 257–8.

Lovett, A. (1985) Community Psychiatry Research Unit, Hackney, in *Good Practices in Mental Health Housing Information Pack*, GPMH, London.

McAusland, T. (1985) Housing for people with long-term psychiatric disabilities – beyond the 24 bedded unit?, in *Good Practices in Mental Health Housing Information Pack*, GPMH, London.

MacCarthy, B. (1988) The Role of Relatives, in *Community Care in Practice: Services for the Continuing Care Client*, (eds A. Lavender and F. Holloway), Wiley, Chichester, pp. 207–30.

McCowan, P. and Wilder, H. (1975) *Lifestyle of 100 Psychiatric Patients*, Psychiatric Rehabilitation Association, London.

McDougall, S. (1992) The effect of nutritional education on the shopping and eating habits of a small group of chronic schizophrenic patients living in the community. *British Journal of Occupational Therapy*, **558**(2), 62–8.

Mahoney, J. (1988) Finance and government policy, in *Community Care in Practice: Services for the Continuing Care Client*, (eds A. Lavender and F. Holloway), Wiley, Chichester, pp. 75–90.

Mann, S.A. and Cree, W. (1976) New long-stay psychiatric patients: a national sample survey of fifteen mental hospitals in England and Wales 1972/3. *Psychological Medicine*, **6**(4), 603–16.

Mechanic, D. (1986) The challenge of chronic mental illness: a retrospective and prospective view. *Hospital and Community Psychiatry*, **37**(9), 891–6.

Meteyard, B. (1990) *The Community Care Keyworker Manual*, Longman, London.

Miller, N. (1988) The informal care network, in *Integrating Care Systems*, (ed. D. Stockford), Longman, London.

MIND (1990) *Advocacy: Different forms of Empowerment*, MIND, London.

Mosher, L.R. and Burti, L. (1989) *Community Mental Health: Principles and Practice*, Norton, New York.

Murdoch, A. (1988) Skills mix. *British Journal of Occupational Therapy*, **51**(2), 37.

Murdock, C. (1992) A critical evaluation of the Barthel Index, Part 1. *British Journal of Occupational Therapy*, **55**(3), 109–11.

Murray, J. (1978) *Special Housing?*, MIND, London.

Nader, R. (ed.) (1973) *The Consumer and Corporate Accountability*, Harcourt Brace Jovanovich, New York.

National Schizophrenia Fellowship (1979) *Home Sweet Nothing*, National Schizophrenia Fellowship, London.

Nisbet, R. (1985) Community accommodation project, Leicester, in *Good Practices in Mental Health Housing Information Pack*, GPMH, London.

Norris, R. (1989) New Horizons. *British Journal of Occupational Therapy*, **52**(5), 188–93.

Olsen, M.R. (1979) Boarding out and substitute family care of the psychiatric patient, in *The Care of the Mentally Disordered: An examination of Some Alternatives to Hospital Care*, (ed. M.R. Olsen), British Association of Social Workers, Birmingham.

Onyett, S. (1992) *Case Management in Mental Health*, Chapman and Hall, London.

Ovretveit, J. (1989) *Essentials of Multi-Professional Community Team Organisation*, Brunel Institute of Organisation and Social Studies, Uxbridge.

Patmore, C. and Weaver, T. (1991) *Community Mental Health Teams: Lessons for Planners and Managers*, GPMH, London.

Pilling, S. (1988) Work and the continuing care client, in *Community Care in Practice: Services for the Continuing Care Client*, (eds A. Lavender and F. Holloway), Wiley, Chichester, pp. 75–90.

Pilling, S. (1991) *Rehabilitation and Community Care*, Routledge, London.

Ramon, S. (1988) Community Care in Britain, in *Community*

Care in Practice: Services for the Continuing Care Client, (eds A. Lavender and F. Holloway), Wiley, Chichester, pp. 9–26.

Rapp, C.A. (1988) *The Strengths Perspective of Case Management with Persons Suffering from Severe Mental Illness*, NIMH, University of Kansas.

Rapp, C.A. and Kisthardt, W.E. (1991) Bridging the gap between principles and practice, in *Case Management and Social Work Practice*, (ed. S.M. Rose), Longman, New York.

Rapp, C.A. and Wintersteen, R. (1989) The Strengths Model of Case Management: results from twelve demonstrations. *Psychosocial Rehabilitation Journal*, **13**(1), 23–32.

Reed, K.L. (1984) *Models of Practice in Occupational Therapy*, Williams and Wilkins, Baltimore.

Reid, J. (1988) Community care: combining knowledge. *British Journal of Occupational Therapy*, **51**(11), 375.

Renshaw, J. (1987) The challenge of enabling the client to be a consumer. *Social Work Today* 27/7/87, 10–11.

Richter, D. (ed.) (1984) *Research in Mental Illness*, Heinemann, London.

Robson, G. (1987) Nagging: models of advocacy, in *Power in Strange Places*, (eds I. Barker and E. Peck), GPMH, London.

Rosen, A., Hadzi-Pavlovic, D. and Parker, G. (1989) The life skills profile: a measure assessing function and disability in schizophrenia. *Schizophrenia Bulletin*, **15**(2), 325–37.

Rowland, M. (1990) *Rights Guide to Non-means-tested Benefits*, (13th edn), Child Poverty Action Group, Great Britain.

Ryan, P. (1979) Residential care for the mentally disabled, in *Community Care for the Mentally Disabled*, (eds J.K. Wing and R. Olsen), Oxford University Press, Oxford.

Ryan, P., Ford, R. and Clifford, P. (1991) *Case Management and Community Care*, Research and Development for Psychiatry, London.

Segal, S.P. and Moyles, E.W. (1979) Management style and institutional dependency in sheltered care. *Social Psychiatry*, **14**, 159–65.

Shamash, J. (1991) Poor cows, *Midweek* magazine 14/11/91, 12–14.

Shepherd, G. (1988a) Evaluation and service planning, in *Community Care in Practice: Services for the Continuing Care Client*, (eds A. Lavender and F. Holloway), Wiley, Chichester, pp. 91–114.

Shepherd, G. (1988b) Psychological interventions in the treatment of schizophrenia, in *Schizophrenia: The Major Issues* (eds P. Bebbington and P. McGuffin), Heinemann, Oxford, pp. 226–43.

Shepherd, G. (1990) Case management. *Health Trends*, **22**(2), 59–61.

Shepherd, G. (1991) Foreword, in *Theory and Practice of Psychiatric Rehabilitation*, 3rd edn, (eds F.N. Watts and D.H. Bennett), Churchill Livingstone, Edinburgh.

Shepherd, M., Cooper, B., Brown, A.C. and Kalton, G. (1981) *Psychiatric Illness in General Practice*, 2nd edn, Oxford University Press, Oxford.

Social Services Committee (1985) *Community Care with Special Reference to Adult Mentally Ill and Mentally Handicapped People*, HMSO, London.

Stein, L. and Test, M.A. (1980) Alternatives to mental hospital treatment. *Archives of General Psychiatry*, **37**, 392–7.

Szasz, T.S. (1961) *The Myth of Mental Illness*, Harper & Row, New York.

Tarrier, N. (1990) The family management of schizophrenia, in *Reconstructing Schizophrenia*, (ed. R.P. Bentall), Routledge, London.

Tarrier, N. (1991) Behavioural psychotherapy and schizophrenia. *Behavioural Psychotherapy*, **19**(1), 121–30.

Tarrier, N., Barrowclough, C., Proceddu, K. and Watts, S. (1988a) The assessment of psychophysiological reactivity to the expressed emotion of the relatives of schizophrenic patients. *British Journal of Psychiatry*, **152**, 618–24.

Tarrier, N., Barrowclough, C., Vaughn, C. *et al.* (1988b) The community management of schizophrenia: a controlled trial of a behavioural intervention with families to reduce relapse. *British Journal of Psychiatry*, **153**, 532–42.

Thorner, S. (1991) The essential skills of an occupational therapist. *British Journal of Occupational Therapy*, **54**(6), 222–3.

Timms, P.W. and Fry, A.H. (1989) Homelessness and mental illness.

Health Trends, **21**, 70–1.

Trombly, C. (ed. (1989) *Occupational Therapy for Physical Dysfunction*, 3rd edn, Williams and Wilkins, Baltimore.

Vaughan, P.J. (1985) Developments in psychiatric day care. *British Journal of Psychiatry*, **147**, 1–4.

Vaughan, P.J. and Prechner, M. (1986) A structured approach to psychiatric day care. *British Journal of Occupational Therapy* **49**(1), 10–12.

Vostanis, P. (1990) The Role of Work in Psychiatric Rehabilitation: a Review of the Literature. *British Journal of Occupational Therapy*, **53**(1), 24–8.

Wansborough, N. (1981) The place of work in rehabilitation, in *Handbook of Psychiatric Rehabilitation Practice*, (eds J.K. Wing and B. Morris), Oxford University Press, Oxford.

Warner, R. (1985) *Recovery from Schizophrenia*, Routledge and Kegan Paul, Boston.

Watts, F.N. and Bennett, D.H. (eds) (1991) *Theory and Practice of Psychiatric Rehabilitation*, 3rd edn, Churchill Livingstone, Edinburgh.

Weick, A., Rapp, C., Patrick Sullivan, W. and Kisthardt, W. (1989) A strengths perspective for social work practice. *Social Work*, **33**, 350–4.

Williams, J. and Watson, G. (1988) Sexual inequality, family life and family therapy, in *Family Therapy in Britain* (eds. E. Street and W. Dryden), Open University Press, Milton Keynes.

Willie, C.V., Kramer, B.M. and Brown, B.S. (1973) *Racism and Mental Health*, University of Pittsburgh Press.

Willis, J. (1984) *Lecture Notes on Psychiatry*, 6th edn, Blackwell Scientific Publications, Oxford.

Willson, M. (1984) *Occupational Therapy in Short-term Psychiatry*, Churchill Livingstone, Edinburgh.

Wilson, M. (1987) *Occupational Therapy in Long-term Psychiatry*, 2nd edn, Churchill Livingstone, Edinburgh.

Wing, J.K. (ed.) (1982) Long-term community care: experience in a London borough. *Psychological Medicine Monograph Supplement*, **2**.

Wing, J.K. and Brown, G. (1970) *Institutionalisation and Schizophrenia*, Cambridge, University Press, Cambridge.

Wing, J.K. and Morris, B. (eds) (1981) *Handbook of Psychiatric Practice*, Oxford University Press, Oxford.

Witheridge, T.F. (1989) The assertive community treatment worker: an emerging role and its implications for professional training. *Hospital and Community Psychiatry*, 40(6), 620–4.

Wykes, T. (1982) A hostel-ward for new long-stay patients in long-term community care (ed. J.K. Wing), *Psychological Medicine Monograph Supplement*, 2.

Further reading

Baker, R. and Hall, J.N. (1983) *REHAB: Rehabilitation Evaluation*, Vine Publishing, Aberdeen.

Barrett, J.E. and Rose, R.M. (eds) (1986) *Mental Disorders in the Community*, Guilford Press, New York.

Beardshaw, V. and Towell, D. (1990) *Assessment and case management: implications for the implementation of 'Caring for People'*, Kings Fund Institute Briefing Paper (10), Kings Fund, London.

Bebbington, P. and McGuffin, P. (eds) (1988) *Schizophrenia: The Major Issues*, Heinemann, Oxford.

Bennett, D.H. and Freeman, H.L. (eds) (1991) *Community psychiatry: the principles*, Churchill Livingstone, Edinburgh.

Beynon, S. (1992) Stranger in a strange land: a consumer guide to occupational therapy. *British Journal of Occupational Therapy*, **55**(5), 186–8.

Birchwood, M. and Smith, J. (1985) *Understanding Schizophrenia*, West Birmingham Health Authority Mental Health Services, Birmingham.

Borland, A., McRae, J. and Lycan, C. (1989) Outcomes of five years of intensive care management. *Hospital and Community Psychiatry*, **40**(4), 369–76.

Braisby, D., Echlin, R., Hill, S. and Smith, H. (1988) *Changing Futures: housing and support services for people discharged from psychiatric hospitals*, Kings Fund, London.

Brandon, A. and Brandon, D. (1987) *Consumers as Colleagues*, MIND, London.

Brown, H. and Basset, T. (1988) *First Things First: a Team Building Manual for Community Mental Handicap and Community Mental Health Teams*, South East Thames Regional Health Authority, Bexhill-on-Sea.

Burningham, S. (1989) *Not On Your Own*, Penguin, London.

Butterworth, G. and Skidmore, D. (1981) *Caring for the Mentally Ill in the Community*, Croom Helm, London.

Campbell, A. and McCreadie, R.G. (1983) Occupational therapy is effective for chronic schizophrenic day patients. *British Journal of Occupational Therapy*, **46**(11), 327–8.

Christie, Y. and Blunden, R. (1991) *Is Race on Your Agenda?*, Kings Fund, London.

Davidson, J. (1987) Health education in a psychiatric setting. *British Journal of Occupational Therapy*, **50**(9), 313–15.

Denton, P. (1987) *Psychiatric Occupational Therapy: a workbook of practical skills*, Little Brown, Boston.

Durham, T.M. (1982) Community living skills training in psychiatric rehabilitation. *British Journal of Occupational Therapy*, **45**(7), 233–5.

Echlin, R. (ed) (1988) *Community Mental Health Teams/Centres*, GPMH and Interdisciplinary Asssociation of Mental Health Workers, London.

Echlin, R. (ed) (1990) *Day Care Information Pack*, GPMH, London.

Egan, G. (1986) *The Skilled Helper*, 3rd edn, Brooks/Cole, California.

Fernando, S. (1991) *Mental Health, Race and Culture*, MacMillan, London.

Goering, P.N., Wasylenki, D.A., Farkas, M. *et al.* (1988) What difference does case management make? *Hospital and Community Psychiatry*, **39**(3), 272–6.

Goffman, E. (1961) *Asylums*, Penguin, Harmondsworth.

Goldberg, D. and Huxley, P. (1980) *Mental Illness in the Community: the Pathway to Psychiatric Care*, Tavistock, London.

Good Practices in Mental Health (1985) *Housing Information Pack*, GPMH, London.

Good Practices in Mental Health (1986) *Advocacy Information Pack*, GPMH, London.

Grove, E. (1988) Working Together. *British Journal of Occupational Therapy*, **51**(5), 150–6.

Heginbotham, C. (ed.) (1990) *Caring for People: local strategies for achieving change in community care*, Kings Fund, London.

Henderson, R. and Wallis, M. (1991) *Prisoners, Patients or People?*, Freedom in Action, London.

Holmes, D. (1985) The role of the occupational therapist–work evaluator. *American Journal of Occupational Therapy*, **39**(5), 308–13.

Howell, C. (1986) A controlled trial of goal-setting for long-term community psychiatric patients. *British Journal of Occupational Therapy*, **49**(8), 264–8.

Hume, C. and Pullen, I. (eds) (1986) *Rehabilitation in Psychiatry*, Churchill Livingstone, Edinburgh.

Jenkins, R. (1983) The medical consequences of unemployment. *British Journal of Occupational Therapy*, **46**(8), 220–2.

Johnston, F. and Spratt, G. (1987) Planning ability in schizophrenia: a comparative study. *British Journal of Occupational Therapy*, **50**(9), 309–11.

Kavanagh, D. (ed.) (1992) *Schizophrenia: an overview and practical handbook*, Chapman & Hall, London.

Kielhofner, G. (1985) *A Model of Human Occupation*, Williams and Wilkins, Baltimore.

Kings Fund Centre. (1987) *The Need for Asylum in Society for the Mentally Ill or Infirm*, Kings Fund, London.

Kings Fund Centre (1988) *Action for Carers: A Guide to Multi-disciplinary Support at Local Level*, Kings Fund, London.

Krupa, T., Murphy, M. and Thornton, J. (1988) Treatment of the long-term mentally ill, in *Occupational Therapy in Mental Health*, (eds D. Scott and N. Katz), Taylor and Francis, London.

Lacey, R. (1991) *A Complete Guide to Psychiatric Drugs: A Layman's Handbook*, Ebury Press, London.

Laing, R.D. (1959) *The Divided Self*, Tavistock, London.

Lear, G. and Morris, G. (1991) Case management: the right approach for Roy. *Nursing Times*, **87**(50), 27–8.

Lear, G., Morris, G., Parnell,M. and Wharne, S. (1991) Case management: responding to need. *Nursing Times*, **87**(50), 24–6.

Liberman, R.P. (1988) *Psychiatric Rehabilitation of Chronic Mental Patients*, American Psychiatric Association, Washington.

McIver, S. (1991) *Obtaining the Views of Users of Mental Health Services*, Kings Fund Centre, London.

Markus, A.C., Murray Parkes, C., Tomson, P. and Johnston, M. (1989) *Psychological Problems in General Practice*, Oxford University Press, Oxford.

Martindale, D. (1987) *The CARE System, Working Paper No. 2.*,

National Unit for Psychiatric Research and development, London.

MIND (1986) *Finding Our Own Solutions: Women's Experience of Mental Health Care*, MIND, London.

MIND (1991) *The MIND Guide to Advocacy in Mental Health*, MIND, London.

MIND (1991) *Action Pack on Mental Health and Employment* MIND, London.

Monteath, H. (1983) Work assessment in the current economic climate. *British Journal of Occupational Therapy*, **46**(8), 223–5.

Moss, B.A. (1990) Living Skills Centres: a part of Australia's Community Mental Health Service. *British Journal of Occupational Therapy*, **53**(3), 112–13.

Murphy, E. (1991) *After the Asylums: Community Care for People with Mental Illness*, Faber and Faber, London.

Nathan, J. (1982) Community occupational therapy in the mental health field. *British Journal of Occupational Therapy*, **45**(1), 3–5.

Øvretveit, J. (1992) Concepts of case management. *British Journal of Occupational Therapy*, **55**(6), 225–8.

Pulling, J. (1987) *The Caring Trap*, Fontana, Glasgow.

Rack, P. (1982) Race, Culture and Mental Disorder, Tavistock, London.

Ramon, S. (1987) *Psychiatry in Transition*, Zwan, London.

Ramon, S. (1991) *Beyond Community Care*, MacMillan, London.

Reed, S.M. (1987) Occupational therapists in the interdisciplinary team setting, in *The Changing Roles of Occupational Therapists in the 1980's*, (ed. F.S. Cromwell), Haworth Press, New York.

Renshaw, J. (1987) *The Asylum Trap; What does it mean for mental health care today?*, GPMH, London.

Repper, J. and Peacham, W. (1991) A suitable case for management? *Nursing Times*, **87**(12), 62–5.

Sherman, P.S. and Porter, R. (1991) Mental health consumers as case management aides. *Hospital and Community Psychiatry*, **42**(5), 494–8.

Smith, J. and Birchwood, M. (1990) Relatives and patients as partners in the mangagement of schizophrenia. *British Journal of Psychiatry*, **156**, 654–60.

Spittles, D. (1991) No room for Westminster Homeless, *Observer* newspaper 16/6/91, London.

Survivors Speak Out (1990) *Self Advocacy Action Pack: Empowering Mental Health Service Users.*

Tower Hamlets Mental Health and Housing Working Party (1987) *Stepping Out: Mental Health, Housing and Community Care in Tower Hamlets*, Tower Hamlets Mental Health and Housing Working Party, London.

Trower, P., Bryant, B. and Argyle, M. (1978) *Social Skills and Mental Health*, Methuen, London.

Turner, T. (1988) Community care. *British Journal of Psychiatry*, **152**, 1–3.

Vaughan, P.J. and Prechner, M. (1985) Occupation or therapy in psychiatric day care. *British Journal of Occupational Therapy*, **48**(6), 169–71.

Voisey, P. (1988) Opening a Group Home. *British Journal of Occupational Theapy*, **51**(5), 160–2.

Wertheimer, A. (1989) *Housing: The Foundation of Community Care*, MIND and The National Association of Housing Associations, London.

Wilson, J. (1988) *Caring Together: Guidelines for Carers Self-help and Support Groups*, National Extension College, Cambridge.

Wing, J.K. (1986) Long-term care in schizophrenia: contributions from epidemiologic studies in the United Kingdom, in *Mental Disorders in the Community* (eds J.E. Bennett and R.M. Rose), Guilford Press, New York.

Winn, E. (ed.) (1990) *Power to the People*, Kings Fund, London.

Winn, L. (ed.) (1990) *Power to the People: the Key to Responsive Services in Health and Social Care*, Kings Fund, London.

Woodside, H. (1985) The day centre and its role as a social network. *Hospital and Community Psychiatry*, **36**(2), 177–80.

Bibliography

CHAPTER 1

Barrett, J.E. and Rose, R.M (eds) (1986) *Mental Disorders in the Community*, Guilford Press, New York.

Butterworth, G. and Skidmore, D. (1981) *Caring for the mentally ill in the community*, Croom Helm, London.

Christie, Y. and Blunden, R. (1991) *Is race on your agenda?*, Kings Fund, London.

Davidson, J. (1987) Health Education in a Psychiatric Setting. *British Journal of Occupational Therapy*, **50**(9), 313–15.

Egan, G. (1986) *The Skilled Helper*, 3rd edn, Brooks/Cole, California.

Fernando, S. (1991) *Mental Health, Race and Culture*, MacMillan, London.

Goffman, E. (1961) *Asylums*, Penguin, Harmondsworth.

Goldberg, D. and Huxley, P. (1980) *Mental Illness in the Community: The Pathway to Psychiatric Care*, Tavistock, London.

Heginbotham, C. (ed) (1990) *Caring for People: local strategies for achieving change in community care*, Kings Fund, London.

Hume, C. and Pullen, I. (eds) (1986) *Rehabilitation in Psychiatry*, Churchill Livingstone, Edinburgh.

Kings Fund Centre. (1988) *Action for Carer's: A Guide to Multidisciplinary Support at Local Level*, Kings Fund, London.

Krupa, T., Murphy, M. and Thornton, J. (1988) Treatment of the long-term mentally ill, in *Occupational Therapy in Mental Health*, (eds D. Scott and N. Katz), Taylor and Francis, London.

Liberman, R.P. (1988) *Psychiatric Rehabilitation of Chronic Mental Patients*, American Psychiatric Association, Washington.

MIND (1986) *Finding Our Own Solutions: Women's Experience of Mental Health Care*, MIND, London.

Murphy, E. (1991) *After the Asylums: Community Care for People with Mental Illness*, Faber and Faber, London.

Pulling, J. (1987) *The Caring Trap*, Fontana, Glasgow.

Rack, P. (1982) *Race, Culture and Mental Disorder*, Tavistock, London.

Ramon, S. (1987) *Psychiatry in Transition*, Zwan, London.

Ramon, S. (1991) *Beyond Community Care*, MacMillan, London.

Renshaw, J. (1987) *The Asylum Trap: What does it mean for mental health care today?*, GPMH, London.

Wilson, J. (1988) *Caring Together: Guidelines for Carer's Self- help and Support Groups*, National Extension College, Cambridge.

CHAPTER 2

Beardshaw, V. and Towell, D. (1990) *Assessment and case management: implications for the implementation of 'Caring for People'*, Kings Fund Institute Briefing Paper (10), Kings Fund, London.

Borland, A., McRae, J. and Lycan, C. (1989) Outcomes of five years of intensive case management. *Hospital and Community Psychiatry*, **40**(4), 369–76.

Brown, H. and Bassett, T. (1988) *First Things First: a Team Building Manual for Community Mental Handicap and Community Mental Health Teams*, South East Thames Regional Health Authority, Bexhill-on-Sea.

Echlin, R. (ed) (1988) *Community Mental Health Teams/Centres*, GPMH and Interdisciplinary Association of Mental Health Workers, London.

Goering, P.N., Wasylenki, D.A., Farkas, M. *et al.* (1988) What difference does Case Management make? *Hospital and Community Psychiatry*, **39**(3), 272–76.

Grove, E. (1988) Working Together. *British Journal of Occupational Therapy*, **51**(5), 150–56.

Lear, G. and Morris, G. (1991) Case Management: The Right Approach for Roy. *Nursing Times* **87**(50), 27–28.

Lear, G., Morris, G., Parnell, M. and Wharne, S. (1991) Case Management: Responding to Need. *Nursing Times*, **87**(50), 24–6.

Martindale, D. (1987) The CARE System, Working Paper No. 2., National Unit for Psychiatric Research and Development, London.

Øvretveit, J. (1992) Concepts of Case Management *British Journal of Occupational Therapy*, **55**(6), 225–8.

Reed, S.M. (1987) Occupational therapists in the interdisciplinary team setting, in *The Changing Roles of Occupational Therapists in the 1980's*, (ed. F.S. Cromwell), Haworth Press, New York.

Repper, J. and Peacham, W. (1991) A Suitable Case for Management? *Nursing Times*, **87**(12), 62–5.

Sherman, P.S. and Porter, R. (1991) Mental health consumers as case management aides. *Hospital and Community Psychiatry*, **42**(5), 494–8.

CHAPTER 3

Baker, R. and Hall, J.N. (1983) *REHAB: Rehabilitation Evaluation*, Vine Publishing, Aberdeen.

Howell, C. (1986) A controlled trial of goal-setting for long-term community psychiatric patients. *British Journal of Occupational Therapy*, **49**(8), 264–8.

Kielhofner, G. (1985) *A Model of Human Occupation*, Williams and Wilkins, Baltimore.

CHAPTER 4

Bebbington, P. and McGuffin, P. (eds) (1988) *Schizophrenia: The Major Issues*, Heinemann, Oxford.

Bennett, D.H., Freeman, H.L. (eds) (1991) *Community Psychiatry: the principles*, Churchill Livingstone, Edinburgh.

Birchwood, M. and Smith, J. (1985) *Understanding Schizophrenia*, East Birmingham Health Authority Mental Health Services, Birmingham.

Kavanagh, D. (ed.) (1992) *Schizophrenia: an overview and practical handbook*, Chapman & Hall, London.

Kings Fund Centre. (1987) *The Need for Asylum in Society for the Mentally Ill or Infirm*, Kings Fund, London.

Lacey, R. (1991) *A Complete Guide to Psychiatric Drugs: A Layman's Handbook*, Ebury Press, London.

Laing, R.D. (1959) *The Divided Self*, Tavistock, London.

Markus, A.C., Murray Parkes, C., Tomson, P. and Johnston, M. (1989) *Psychological Problems in General Practice*, Oxford University Press, Oxford.

Smith, J. and Birchwood, M. (1990) Relatives and patients as partners in the management of schizophrenia. *British Journal of Psychiatry*, **156**, 654–60.

Trower, P., Bryant, B. and Argyle, M. (1978) *Social Skills and Mental Health*, Methuen, London.

Turner, T. (1988) Community Care. *British Journal of Psychiatry*, **152**, 1–3.

Wing, J.K. (1986) Long-term Care in Schizophrenia: Contributions from Epidemiologic Studies in the United Kingdom, in *Mental Disorders in the Community*, (eds J.E. Bennett and R.M. Rose), Guilford Press, New York.

CHAPTER 5

Braisby, D., Echlin, R., Hill, S. and Smith, H. (1988) *Changing Futures: housing and support services for people discharged from psychiatric hospitals*, Kings Fund, London.

Good Practices in Mental Health, (1985) *Housing Information Pack*, GPMH, London.

Spittles, D. (1991) No Room for Westminster Homeless, *Observer* newspaper 16/6/91, London.

Tower Hamlets Mental Health and Housing Working Party. (1987) *Stepping Out: Mental Health, Housing and Community Care in Tower Hamlets*, Tower Hamlets Mental Health and Housing Working Party, London.

Voisey, P. (1988) Opening a Group Home. *British Journal of Occupational Therapy*, **51**(5), 160–2.

Wertheimer, A. (1989) *Housing: The Foundation of Community Care*, MIND and the National Association of Housing Associations, London.

CHAPTER 7

Denton, P. (1987) *Psychiatric Occupational Therapy: a workbook of practical skills*, Little Brown, Boston.

Durham, T.M. (1982) Community living skills training in psychiatric rehabilitation. *British Journal of Occupational Therapy*, **45**(7), 233–35.

Johnston, F. and Spratt, G. (1987) Planning Ability in Schizophrenia: a comparative study. *British Journal of Occupational Therapy*, **50**(9), 309–11.

Moss, B.A. (1990) Living Skills Centres: A Part of Australia's Community Mental Health Service. *British Journal of Occupational Therapy*, **53**(3), 112–13.

Nathan, J. (1982) Community Occupational Therapy in the Mental Health Field. *British Journal of Occupational Therapy*, **45**(1), 3–5.

CHAPTER 8

Campbell, A. and McCreadie, R.G. (1983) Occupational therapy is effective for chronic schizophrenic day patients. *British Journal of Occupational Therapy*, **46**(11), 327–8.

Echlin, R. (ed) (1990) *Day Care Information Pack*, GPMH, London.

Holmes, D. (1985) The role of the occupational therapist-work evaluator. *American Journal of Occupational Therapy*, **29**(5), 308–13.

Jenkins, R. (1983) The medical consequences of unemployment. *British Journal of Occupational Therapy*, **46**(8), 220–2.

MIND. (1991) *Action Pack on Mental Health and Employment*, MIND, London.

Monteath, H. (1983) Work assessment in the current economic climate. *British Journal of Occupational Therapy*, **46**(8), 223–5.

Vaughan, P.J. and Prechner, M. (1985) Occupation or therapy in psychiatric day care. *British Journal of Occupational Therapy*, **48**(6), 169–71.

Woodside, H. (1985) The day centre and its role as a social network. *Hospital and Community Psychiatry*, **36**(2), 177–80.

CHAPTER 9

Beynon, S. (1992) Stranger in a Strange Land: A Consumer Guide to Occupational Therapy. *British Journal of Occupational Therapy*, **55**(5), 186–8.

Brandon, A. and Brandon, D. (1987) *Consumers as Colleagues*, MIND, London.

Burningham, S. (1989) *Not On Your Own*, Penguin, London.

Good Practices in Mental Health (1986) *Advocacy Information Pack*, GPMH, London.

Henderson, R. and Wallis, M. (1991) *Prisoners, Patients or People?*, Freedom in Action, London.

McIver, S. (1991) *Obtaining the Views of Users of Mental Health Services*, Kings Fund Centre, London.

MIND. (1990) *The MIND Guide to Advocacy in Mental Health*, MIND, London.

Survivors Speak Out. (1990) *Self Advocacy Action Pack: Empowering Mental Health Service Users.*

Winn, E. (ed) (1990) Power to the People, Kings Fund, London.

Winn, L. (ed) (1990) *Power to the People: The Key to Responsive Services in Health and Social Care*, Kings Fund, London.

Index

Access to Health Records Act (1990) 190
Access to Personal Files Act (1987) 190
Accommodation, see Housing; Sheltered Accommodation
Activities of daily living assessment 150–3
community resources 154–5
core skill 25
definition 141–2
and mental health 153
professional responsibilities 143–4
range 142
see also Personal care
Activity analysis 25, 142–3, 153, 155
Adult education 183
see also Education
Advocacy 8, 127, 138, 184, 186, 188, 192, 194
citizen 193, 210
legal 193
and the mental health professional 96, 118, 119, 126, 197–8, 210
regional and national networks 208–9
self 97, 139, 192, 208, 209–10
see also User empowerment
Appraisals

see also Staff support and supervision
Assessment 53–9
location of 58–9
methods 59
occupational therapy 25
psychiatric symptoms 81–2
timescale of 59
see also Present state examination; Personal strengths model of case management; Occupation
Asset 171
Asylum 67, 70–1
Audit Commission 4
Authority, linked to power 191–2
see also Advocacy; Power

Bed and breakfast 100, 103
see also Board and lodgings; Housing
Befriending schemes 157
Benefits, see Social security benefits
Benefits agency 132, 136
see also Department of Social Security
Bill of Rights, see Patient's Charter; User movement, initiatives
Board and lodgings 100, 115
see also Group homes; Hostels; Housing

Brokerage 37
 model of case management
  33, 35
Budgeting, *see* Finance,
  personal
Burnout 40, 41, 95

Campus community, *see*
  National Schizophrenia
  Fellowship
Care attendant schemes 154–5
Care management 30–1, 32
Care planning 59–61, 62
Care programme 30–1, 32,
  97–8
Carer's 10–11, 112
 relationships with 13, 23–4
 support for 44
 see also Informal care,
  systems of; Psychosocial
  interventions
Caring for People (White
  Paper 1989) 23, 53, 97
Caseload sizes 20, 33, 36, 37
Case management 3, 4, 29–37,
  104, 144, 214
 and assessment 153
 functions of 30–1, 35
 and keyworking 20
 training 37–9, 215
 see also Brokerage model;
  Clinical model; Personal
  strengths model
Case manager 32
 liaison 93–4, 96–7
 monitoring medication 87,
  89
 negotiating with clients 95
 roles and functions 96–8,
  119–20, 138–9, 156, 157,
  184
Case studies 74–6, 109–11,
  130–1, 149–50, 163–6,
  200–3
 see also Personal profiles
Chapter summaries 44–5, 64–5,
  98–9, 121–2, 140, 157–8,
  184–5, 211–2
Chiropody 154

Citizen's advice bureaux 127
Client-centred service 5, 8, 19
Client group 198, 210–11, 213
 characteristics 13–14, 66–7,
  213–4
 definition 11–13
Clinical model of case
  management 33, 35–6
Collaboration
 see also Coordination of
  service functions; Multi-
  disciplinary teams;
  Networking
Community care 1–4, 115,
  216–17
 and carers 10–11
 criticisms 1
 funding 123–5, 216–17
 and the psychiatric hospital
  68–70
 policy for 4
Community centres 155, 157
Community charge, *see* Poll
  Tax
Community Health Council
  191
Community mental health
  centres 2, 181–2
Community mental health
  service
 funding 123–5, 216–17
 organization 20–2
 staffing 18, 21
Community psychiatric nurses
  37, 93, 143–4, 154
Community Psychiatric
  Research Unit 119
Community Yellow Pages, *see*
  User movement,
  initiatives
Consciousness-raising 200,
  203–4
 see also User empowerment;
  User movement
Consumerism 194
Consumer movement 190,
  194
Cooperative employment
  projects 176

Coordination of service
functions 214
see also Monitoring
Core and cluster 116–17
Core skills 19, 24–6, 29, 141,
143, 157
see also Skills mix
Crisis centres, *see* User
movement, initiatives
Crisis houses 120–1
see also Housing, options
and support
Crisis support care, *see* User
movement, initiatives
Counselling, supportive 81, 92

Daily living skills, *see* Activities
of daily living; Personal
care
Data Protection Act (1985) 190
Day care 7–8, 159–60, 173,
176–82
see also Community mental
health centres; Day
centres; Day hospitals
Day centres 2, 177–8
Day hospitals 1, 155–6, 177–8
Debt management 138
see also Finance, personal
Department of Health and
Social Security 132
Department of Health and
Social Security (White
Paper 1975) Better
Services for the Mentally
Ill 177
Department of Social Security
132
Desires, *see* Wants
Dirty squad 154
Disablement Advisory Service
174
Disablement Resettlement
Officer 173
Discharge, *see* Graduated
disengagement
Distribution of financial
resources 7
see also Community mental

health service, funding
District general hospital 1–2, 70
District nurse 90, 120, 154
Domiciliary visit 80, 94–5
Dosett box 89
see also Medication,
monitoring
Dowry system
see also Community mental
health service, funding
Drop-in 157, 178, 179–80, 181
see also Day care; User
movement, initiatives

Early warning signs of relapse
82–3, 153
see also Assessment,
psychiatric symptoms
Education 142, 159, 169, 172,
173, 182–3
of clients and carers 81, 83, 138
Electro convulsive therapy
(ECT) 76, 85, 92–3
Emergency service 95
Employment 159–60
cooperatives 206
interview panels 208
as occupation 166–9
options 173–6
see also Occupation
Employment Act (1944) 174
Employment rehabilitation
centres 175
Engagement 47–53, 139
practical aspects of 50–2
timescale of 49–50
see also Graduated
disengagement;
Relationships with users
Enterprise Allowance Scheme
174
Evaluation 61–4
client involvement 63
see also Monitoring
Expressed emotion 11, 68, 83,
84–5

Family work, *see* Behavioural
interventions

Finance, personal 125–7, 153, 157
  see also Community mental health service, funding
Fountain House, *see* User movement, initiatives

Gender
  issues and mental health 10
General practitioner 7, 9, 93, 94, 95, 96
  and psychiatrist 67–8, 76–8, 89
Graduated disengagement 53
Group homes 101, 104, 114
  see also Hostels; Hostel wards
Group work 81, 156

History-taking 78–81
  see also Monitoring, mental health; Present state examination
Home help organizers 154
Home helps 120, 154, 157
Homelessness and mental health 102–4
Homeless person's unit 103, 118
Hospital casualty department 80
Hospital, mental, *see* Psychiatric hospital
Hostels 100–1, 102, 111, 113–4
  see also Group homes; Housing; Hostel wards
Hostel wards 70, 104,, 113
House of Commons Social Services Committee (1985) 97, 100, 117
Housing
  allocation and management 117–20
  and mental health 104–6, 119
  options and support 7, 100–2, 111–21
  ordinary 117–20
  see also User movement, initiatives

Housing Act (1985) 103
Housing Associations 119
  see also Housing, ordinary

Industrial Therapy Organization 174
Informal care, systems of 23, 155
  see also Carers
Informal support for staff 43–4
  see also Staff support and supervision
Information-sharing with users 92, 190–1, 194
  legal rights 204
Institutional living patterns 3
Institutions
  affects of 1
  see also Psychiatric hospitals, closure

Job centres 173–4
Job clubs 174
Job descriptions 42
  see also Staff support and supervision
Job Start allowance 174
Joint finances 124
  see also Community mental health services, funding

Keyworker 27–9, 32, 178, 198
  see also Multi-disciplinary teams; Uni-disciplinary teams
Kings Fund College 125
Kirkdale Resource Centre 181

Lambeth Accord Worklink 171
Lambeth Link Self Advocacy Project 206, 207, 208, 209, 218–21
  see also User empowerment; User movement
Laundry service 154
Legal 204
  see also Legislative issues; Litigation
Legislative issues 96–8

Leisure 142, 159, 160, 169, 173, 182–3
Life events 68, 83–4, 104
Life Skills Profile 151
    see also Activities of daily living, assessment
Line management 23, 28, 39–40, 41–2
    see also Staff support and supervision
Litigation 8, 190
    see also Legal
Lunatic asylum, *see* Asylum

Meals-on-wheels 120, 154, 157
Medical model 7, 22, 47–8, 67, 76, 81–2, 85
    biopsychosocial 78
Medication 1, 68, 76, 77, 85–92
    administration 25, 86–7
    information 207
    maintenance 87–8
    monitoring 88–90, 96
    objections to 90–2
    overdose 89–90
    polypharmacy 91
    side-effects 87, 90–1
    see also Tardive Dyskinesia
Mental Health Act (1983) 96, 97
    detention 25, 71, 92, 96, 97
Mental Health User's Centre 179–80
Mental illness specific grant 125
    see also Community mental health service, funding
Mental Patients Association 179
    see also User movement, initiative
Mill, The 179
Minister for Social Security 135
Monitoring 28, 61
    early warning signs 82–3
    medication 88–90
    mental health 78–82
    see also Coordination of service functions; Evaluation

Multi-disciplinary teams 18–19, 26, 104
    and the case manager 29–37
    in hospital settings 21
    and keyworking 27–9
    planning and management 40
    staff joint working 43
    and teamwork 19
    see also Uni-disciplinary teams

National Foundation of Patients Advocates (Holland) 193
National Schizophrenia Fellowship 112
Needs 13, 18, 186, 192, 213
    areas of 6–8, 100, 101, 103, 167
    assessment 54–8, 104–6, 151–2
    and engagement 49
    meeting of 4–5, 6, 95, 117–21, 139, 154–5, 159, 177–81, 188–9, 197

Networking 23, 93–4
    see also Brokerage
Nursing homes 100–1, 115
    see also Hostels

Occupation 166–9
    assessment and rehabilitation 169–73
    see also Employment
Occupational counselling 169, 170, 176
Occupational therapists 58, 151, 176, 179, 184
Occupational therapy 88, 154, 155–6, 171, 172, 215
    and client needs 29, 34–5
    core skills 24–6, 141, 143, 150, 157
    models for practice 46–7
    and policy-making 26

Occupational therapy (*contd*)
  problem-solving 47, 54, 60
  process 6, 47, 61
Operational policies 42, 196
Out of hours services 180–81
Outreach 36, 48, 104, 169, 214

Patients Charter 209, 218–21
  see also Lambeth Link Self
    Advocacy Project
Patient councils 205
  see also User empowerment;
    User movement
Personal care 7–8, 143, 153,
    154, 157
  see also Activities of daily
    living
Personal profiles 14–17, 71–4,
    107–9, 127–30, 145–9,
    161–3
  see also Case studies
Personal strengths model of
    case management 4, 33,
    35–6, 47, 53, 135, 156,
    214–15
  and assessment 55–8
  and care planning 61, 62
  and engagement 48
  principles of 33–4
Pharmacist 89
Physical illness 13, 102
  and health promotion
    8–9
Physiotherapy 154
Pill mill 89
  see also Dosett box;
    Medication, monitoring
Poll Tax 51, 133
Power 67, 68, 78, 151, 186,
    189–91, 194–6
Practical skills 155–7
  see also Training
Present state examination
    78–81
  see also History-taking;
    Monitoring, mental
    health
Prison 100, 103
Providers of support 20–4

Psychiatric hospital 70–1, 100
  closure 2, 76
  and community care 68–70
  financial costs 2, 123–5
Psychiatric out-patient clinic
    80, 94, 179–80
Psychiatric Rehabilitation
    Association
  restaurant club 180
Psychiatric ward 80, 104, 113,
    151, 205
Psychiatrist 7, 9, 93–8,
    207
  and care programming 31–2
  and diagnosis 77–81
  and the General Practitioner
    67–8, 76–8, 89
  and multi-disciplinary teams
    22
Psychologists 151
Psychosocial interventions 7,
    68, 82–5, 93
Psychosurgery 76
Psychotherapy 34, 88

Race and culture 9–10
Refuge, *see* Asylum
Rehabilitation 104, 138
  functional skills 76–7
  occupational 171–3
Relationships with users 4–5,
    25–6, 34–5, 36, 153,
    160
  difficulties establishing 6,
    13, 214
  see also Engagement
Remploy 174
Research and development
    for Psychiatry (RDP)
    38
Resettlement and rehabilitation
    112
Resettlement worker, *see*
    Special needs
    resettlement teams
Restart interview, *see*
    Employment, options;
    Job centres
Retreat, *see* Asylum

Role-blurring 22, 25
  and loss of identity 25
  see also Core skills; Multi-
    disciplinary teams; Skills
    mix

Safe house, *see* Asylum
Schizophrenia, symptoms of
  66–7
  see also Client group
Secretary of State for Social
  Security 135
Self-determination 1, 49, 101–2
  see also Personal strengths
    model of case manage-
    ment, principles of
Self-disclosure 52
Sheltered accommodation
  114–15
  see also Housing
Sheltered employment 159–60,
  166, 173, 174–5
  see also Employment,
    options
Sheltered individual placement
  schemes 175–6
  see also Employment,
    options
Skillnet 171
Skills mix 19
  see also Core skills
Skills training, *see* practical
  skills; Training
Slang 12
Social Fund 133, 135–6, 137
  see also Social security
    benefits
Social security benefits 125,
  127, 132–5, 182
  disagreement with decisions
    135
  methods of payment 136–7
  see also Department of Social
    Security; Finance
Social security system 7, 101,
  132–8
Social therapy 88
Social workers 37, 95, 113,
  137, 139, 143

Special needs resettlement
  teams 117–18
  see also Housing, ordinary
Staff support and supervision
  20, 23, 36, 39–44
Stigma 11, 167, 188, 204, 206
Stress vulnerability model 8
Suicide potential 90
Support staff 20, 23, 39
  see also Providers of
    support

Tardive dyskinesia 87, 88, 91
  see also Medication
Tardive psychosis 88
Team planning days 42
  see also Staff support and
    supervision
Therapeutic earnings 174
Training 142, 159, 215
  practical skills 155–7
  user involvement 209–10
  see also Education;
    Occupation; User
    movement, initiatives

Uni-disciplinary teams 25–6,
  28, 36
  and core skills 24
  see also Multi-disciplinary
    teams
User empowerment 8, 50, 186,
  188, 194–6, 216–17
  and the mental health
    professional 194, 196–200
  see also Advocacy
User movement 8, 96, 188,
  210, 215–16
  historical development 187
  initiatives 120, 139, 175–6,
    179, 203–10, 218–21

Voluntary services 95, 101,
  121, 124, 154–5, 176–7,
  179–80
  and work assessment 170,
    171
Voluntary work 166, 172, 174,
  176

Wants 18, 106, 139, 159, 194–5,
    213–14
  assessment 55
  see also Needs
Welfare benefits, *see* Social
    security benefits

Welfare rights adviser 139
Work, *see* Employment;
    Occupation
Working partnership, *see*
    Relationships with
    users